American Health Care Today

And Its Providers

American Health Care Today And Its Providers

by

Linda Hewitt

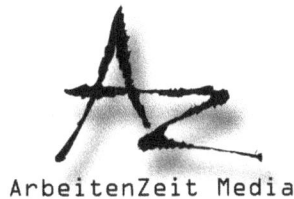

ArbeitenZeit Media

American Health Care Today And Its Providers

ISBN 10 Kindle Edition: 1-941168-28-0
ISBN 13 Kindle Edition: 978-1-941168-28-8
ISBN 10 Trade Paperback Edition: 1-941168-27-2
ISBN 13 Trade Paperback Edition: 978-1-941168-27-1
ISBN 10 Hardback Edition: 1-941168-29-9
ISBN 13 Hardback Edition: 978-1-941168-29-5

Library of Congress Control Number: 2017905998

LEGAL DISCLAIMER

AN ORIGINAL WORK
American Health Care Today And Its Providers

is an original work of nonfiction by Linda Hewitt (2017 May 21)

THANKS

*To the corporate clients whose communications projects began my professional
interest in American health care and what it takes to support it
and to the physicians whose efforts have delivered the benefits
of today's health care to me and my family
and whose information has enriched my understanding
of some of the issues involved, particularly
Charles Simonton, M.D., FACC, FSCAI, then of the Sanger Heart Clinic in
Charlotte, NC, and now Chief Medical Officer and Divisional Vice President of
Medical Affairs for Abbott's vascular division;
Kevin D. Brown, M.D., PhD, Associate Professor, UNC Otolaryngology/Head and
Neck Surgery and Chief of Division of Otology/Neurotology, Skull Base Surgery;
and Matthew G. Ewend, M.D., FACS, Chair of the Department of Neurosurgery
at UNC, President, UNC Faculty Physicians, and Chief Quality and Value
Officer, UNC Health Care.*

*And most especially to the late Drs. Sherrill, Hobbs & Sherrill,
then-eminent orthopedic surgeons of Birmingham, Alabama,
who gave me at the age of seventeen my first adult job
and allowed me to observe the life-enhancing difference made
by talented, committed physicians practicing state-of-the-art medicine.*

CONTENTS

PART ONE. AMERICAN HEALTH CARE TODAY

PART TWO. THE PROVIDER UNIVERSE

Seventeen. Major Challenge: The Political-Football Factor — 104

Eighteen. Physicians Caught In A Perfect Storm — 111

Nineteen. Hospitals Having A Challenging Day — 137

Twenty-Three. Typical Health Episode

Today & Tomorrow   191

Twenty-Four. Dream, Promise & Likely Reality   199

APPENDICES

APPENDIX A. Acronyms Used In This Book   203

APPENDIX B. Useful Online Resources: A Selection   210

PREVIEW   247

SUCCESSFUL PATIENT: Step-By-Step Strategies To Get The Health Care You Need by Linda Hewitt

Chapter One. No One Expects The Unexpected

PART ONE.
AMERICAN
HEALTH CARE
TODAY

Chapter One.

The Purpose Of This Book

The purpose of this book is to provide an overview of U.S. health and health care in 2017.

The first part of the book looks at health care in general: where we get it; who provides it; what it costs and who pays; why it costs so much; who regulates, legislates, and influences it; its scope and nature; the miracles it performs; medical errors and failures; and the outcomes for patients, providers, and payers.

The second part of the book moves into The Provider Universe, that conglomeration of doctors, nurses, hospitals, and all the other occupations and entities that make up the American health-care industry. We take an up-close look at major challenges facing providers, including medical advances and new technology, information technology, emerging care-delivery models, new reimbursement practices, patient empowerment, and politics. We examine how these challenges and others are affecting three key players in The Provider Universe: doctors; nurses; and hospitals.

The third part of the book anticipates what the changing Provider Universe means for patients and how it is likely to affect care.

Health care represents a dichotomy, a "mom and apple pie" issue that can become controversial in a heartbeat. The book is not an attempt to glorify The Provider Universe (in spite of the fact that its work is often glorious), nor is it a statement of blame (in spite of the industry's well-publicized mistakes). I'm a fan, but of the "seen too much to think it's perfect" variety. Rather, this is a brief examination of what's going on with an occasional nod toward "why," an informed observer's excursion into one of the most-important segments of American business.

In short, this is not a book of policy, advocacy, or espousing of any particular political, economic, or sociological position. Nor is it a book that includes the specifics of Medicare, Medicaid, or employer or insurance-company health plans. Nor is it a book arguing for either technological advances or a return to "back in the day" care. Rather, it is about the nature of health care in America today, what it takes to deliver it, and some of the tradeoffs involved.

My approach has been to present information drawn from reliable sources in order to "paint a picture" of this remarkably complicated topic. For some years

I've written about health, health care, safety, and related economic issues for corporate clients and also devised strategy for award-winning communications campaigns relating to health and environmental issues. My recent personal experience as both patient and advocate triggered my interest in learning more about American health care from the patient's perspective and led me to share what I've learned.

My aim is to produce a readable, non-technical introduction to this topic that affects all of us so profoundly. At the conclusion of the book, there are two appendices, one containing a list of acronyms and the other a list of online resources concerning various health-related topics.

Chapter Two.

Where We Get Health Care

Today, we get health care in a wide range of settings.

Doctors' offices remain the primary destination for most of us when we feel ill, need to monitor a condition, want an annual physical, or have another non-urgent medical need. Typically, an appointment is required to see a doctor, and this must usually be made days or weeks in advance. Often, even with an appointment, patients must wait past the expected time.

Other ambulatory care facilities — i.e., facilities offering medical services performed on an outpatient basis so that patients are treated without being admitted to a hospital or other facility — include: dialysis clinics; ambulatory surgical centers; hospital outpatient departments; and offices of health professionals.

Urgent-care centers are a particular type of ambulatory care — walk-in clinics that assist patients with an illness or injury that, while not life-threatening, requires rapid medical attention.

Hospitals offer various services, inpatient and outpatient, that require overnight stays, anesthesia, and/or the use of sophisticated diagnostic and surgical equipment. There are many kinds of hospitals, some limited to specific populations (prisoners, students, the military, and the like). The general public has access to what the American Hospital Association (AHA) terms "community" hospitals. The "community" category includes facilities that range from small local hospitals, large safety-net hospitals, and regional medical centers, to teaching hospitals.

Hospital emergency rooms are intended to handle life-threatening situations or conditions too immediately serious and complex to be addressed by urgent-care centers.

Post-acute care addresses the needs of patients no longer requiring hospital stays but not ready to return to a home setting without aid. Post-acute settings include long-term-care hospitals, inpatient rehabilitation facilities, and skilled nursing facilities. Home health agencies are also listed in this classification.

Hospices provide end-of-life care and/or services in either the patient's home or a physical facility operated by the hospice.

Pharmacies dispense drugs, both prescription and non-prescription.

Ambulance services — ground, air, and water — provide medical transport.

Other settings in which we get care include employer clinics, the offices of school nurses, and similar occupational and educational environments.

The bottom line on where we get health care is that, increasingly, we seek out purpose-specific providers. That's because they tend to be simpler to access, quicker to address our needs, and less expensive.

Chapter Three.

Who Provides Health Care?

Physicians are just the tip of the medical-occupation iceberg. The Henry J. Kaiser Family Foundation estimates that as of May 2014, over twelve million people were employed in health care in the United States, not including certain self-employed individuals. Other sources put the figure as high as sixteen million.

According to the 2016-2017 *Occupational Outlook Handbook (OOH)* issued by the U.S. Department of Labor (DOL) / U.S. Bureau of Labor Statistics (BLS), here — in order of the numbers employed — are the employment statistics for various health-care fields in 2014:

◊   *Registered Nurses - 2,751,000*

◊   *Nursing Assistants and Orderlies - 1,545,200*

◊   *Home Health Aides - 913,500*

◊   *Licensed Practical and Licensed Vocational Nurses - 719,900*

◊   *Physicians and Surgeons - 708,300*

◊   *Medical Assistants - 591,300*

◊   *Pharmacy Technicians - 372,500*

◊   *Dental Assistants - 318,800*

◊   *Medical and Clinical Laboratory Technologists and Technicians - 328,200*

◊   *Pharmacists - 297,100*

◊   *EMTs and Paramedics - 241,200*

◊   *Radiologic and MRI Technologists - 230,600*

◊   *Physical Therapists - 210,900*

◊ Dental Hygienists - 200,500

◊ Medical Records and Health Information Technicians - 188,600

◊ Nurse Anesthetists, Nurse Midwives, and Nurse Practitioners - 170,400

◊ Massage Therapists - 168,800

◊ Dentists - 151,500

◊ Psychiatric Technicians and Aides - 145,200

◊ Speech-Language Pathologists - 135,400

◊ Physical Therapist Assistants and Aides - 128,700

◊ Respiratory Therapists - 120,700

◊ Occupational Therapists - 114,600

◊ Diagnostic Medical Sonographers and Cardiovascular Technologists and Technicians, including Vascular Technologists - 112,700

◊ Phlebotomists - 112,700

◊ Surgical Technologists - 99,800

◊ Veterinary Technologists and Technicians - 95,600

◊ Physician Assistants - 94,400

◊ Veterinarians - 78,300

◊ Opticians, Dispensing - 75,200

◊ Veterinary Assistants and Laboratory Animal Caretakers - 73,400

◊ Occupational Health and Safety Specialists - 70,300

◊ Medical Transcriptionists - 70,000

◊ Dietitians and Nutritionists - 66,700

◊ Chiropractors - 45,200

◊ Occupational Therapy Assistants and Aides - 41,900

◊ Optometrists - 40,600

◊ *Athletic trainers - 25,400*

◊ *Nuclear Medicine Technologists - 20,700*

◊ *Recreational Therapists - 18,600*

◊ *Radiation Therapists - 16,600*

◊ *Exercise Physiologists - 14,500*

◊ *Occupational Health and Safety Technicians - 15,100*

◊ *Audiologists - 13,200*

◊ *Podiatrists - 9,600*

◊ *Orthotists and Prosthetists - 8,300*

◊ *Genetic Counselors - 2,400*

Most of these occupations have specific and sometimes extensive educational requirements and demand some form of licensing or registration. Median pay in 2014 was all over the place. Home health aides, for example, third most numerous health-care occupation according to the BLS, typically need few educational credentials, are not licensed, and have a median pay of $21,380 per year or $10.28 per hour. Registered nurses (RNs), first most numerous, usually have a bachelor of nursing degree from an accredited institution, are licensed, and have a median pay of $66,640 per year or $32.04 per hour. Going along the food chain, physicians and surgeons, fifth most numerous, must hold the MD degree and have completed all intern, residency, and fellowship requirements for their specialty, are licensed, and have a median pay of $187,200 per year or $90.00 per hour.

This list of the occupations broken out by the *OOH* demonstrates the range of health-care positions, as well as confirms the importance of health care as an employing industry, which explains how the medical system gets some of its political clout — that's a lot of voters.

Overall, the health-care industry appears to be doing a good job of convincing the public of the quality of its practitioners. Each year, Gallup polls a representative sampling of Americans to see which professions are held to be the most honest and ethical. In the poll released in December 2016, members of the health-care industry occupied the top three places: nurses, with an 84% "very high/high" rating; pharmacists with a 67% rating; and medical doctors with a 65% rating.

Chapter Four.

What Health Care Costs, Who Pays & For What

Centers for Medicare and Medicaid Services (CMS) numbers for 2014, interpreted by Josh Cothran, Georgia Institute of Technology, in "US Health Care Spending: Who Pays?," (California Health Care Foundation, December 2015) indicate that over two-and-a-half trillion dollars was spent on health care in the U.S.

Categories Of Health-Care Expenditure

◊   *38% - $971.8 billion on "hospital care"*

◊   *24%, - $603.7 billion on "physician and clinical services"*

◊   *12% - $297.7 billion on "prescription drugs"*

◊   *6% - $155.6 billion on "nursing care facilities"*

◊   *6% - $150.4 billion on "other health care"*

◊   *4% - $113.5 billion on "dental services"*

◊   *4% - $103.3 billion on "other medical products"*

◊   *3% - $84.4 billion on "other professional services"*

◊   *3% - $83.2 billion on "home health care"*

Who Pays For Health Care In The U.S.?

There are basically six sources of funding:

◊   *Out-of-pocket — This is the individual consumer paying for uninsured health-care expenses, as well as for deductibles and co-pays.*

◊   *Private insurance — This includes private companies issuing health-insurance policies.*

◊   *Medicare — This is the federal health-insurance program for* people 65 or older, certain younger people with disabilities, and people with End-Stage Renal Disease (permanent kidney failure requiring dialysis or a transplant).

◊ Medicaid – This is the jointly funded, federal-state health-insurance program for low-income and needy people, covering children, the aged, blind, and/or disabled and other people eligible to receive federally assisted income maintenance payments.

◊ Other public insurance – This is insurance coverage written by government bodies or operated by private agencies under government supervision and control (not including Medicare and Medicaid).

◊ Other payers –This includes any health-care payers not listed above, such as self-funded employer plans or medical reimbursement programs.

Here's what each of these funding sources paid for health care in 2014:

◊ $867.9 billion was paid by private insurance – Two biggest categories of expenditure were $361.1 billion for "hospital care" and $254.7 billion for "physician and clinical services."

◊ $680.7 billion was paid by Medicare –Two biggest categories of expenditure were $250.3 billion for "hospital care" and $238.4 billion for "physician and clinical services."

◊ $444.9 billion was paid by Medicaid – Two biggest categories of expenditure were $168.0 billion for "hospital care" and $83.9 billion for "other health care."

◊ $105.9 billion was paid by other public insurance – Two biggest categories of expenditure were $60.4 billion for "hospital care" and $25.2 billion for "physician and clinical services."

◊ $329.9 billion was paid out-of-pocket – Two biggest categories of expenditure were $78.3 billion for "other medical products" and $54.0 billion for "physician and clinical services."

◊ $233.6 billion was paid by other payers – Two biggest categories of expenditure were $99.7 billion for "hospital care" and $67.4 billion for "physician and clinical services."

Who were the big spenders in each category?

◊ *"Hospital care" — Private insurance paid 37%, or $361.1 billion.*

◊ *"Physician and clinical services" — Private insurance paid 42%, or $254.7 billion.*

◊ *"Prescription drugs" — Private insurance paid 43%, or $127.3 billion.*

◊ *"Nursing care facilities" — Medicaid paid 32%, or $49.6 billion.*

◊ *"Other health care" — Medicaid paid 56%, or $83.9 billion.*

◊ *"Dental services" — Private insurance paid 48%, or $54.1 billion.*

◊ *"Home health care" — Medicare paid 42%, or $34.7 billion.*

◊ *"Other medical products" — Out-of-pocket paid 76%, or $78.3 billion.*

◊ *"Other professional services" — Private insurance paid 35%, or $29.7 billion.*

Private insurance was the big spender in five of these categories, demonstrating its ongoing importance in health care.

Which Category Of Payer Will Increase?

Medicare's importance will grow as Baby Boomers, born 1946 through 1964, age into coverage, and the last of the Boomers won't reach the current eligibility age of sixty-five until 2029 even as life expectancy remains relatively constant or increases for those seniors already covered.

The most noticeable trend here, however, will probably be the ongoing growth of out-of-pocket expenditures that will, to one extent or another, be borne by all ages of patients. This will be due to (1) increases in co-pays and deductibles imposed by employer health plans trying to offset exploding premium costs; (2) high-deductible plans purchased by bargain hunters buying their own coverage and seeking the lowest premium; (3) payment for unreimbursable medical services and products, such as cosmetic surgery, most forms of massage, hearing aids, eye glasses, contact lenses, and experimental treatment; (4) price increases by pharmaceutical companies for drugs that aren't fully covered by insurance formularies; (5) increasing difficulty of finding all the medical services necessary for a health event within the patient's insurance-plan network and having to pay more to go outside the network; and (6) payment for health-related gear not covered by insurance, such as exercise equipment, eHealth devices, and the like.

How We Spend Health-Care Money

A study published in the *Journal of the American Medical Association (JAMA)* in 2016 provides some interesting insights.

◊ *Chronic diseases, many preventable, are expensive. The three costliest diseases in 2013 were diabetes ($101 billion); the most common form of heart disease ($88 billion); and back and neck pain ($88 billion).*

◊ *There's no uniformity in yearly spending increases according to disease. In the two decades covered by the study, costs associated with diabetes and low back and neck pain grew much faster than overall spending, while heart-disease spending grew at a slower rate.*

◊ *Once past babyhood, as people age they generally consume more medical resource than they did when they were younger.*

◊ *Spending on public health and prevention does not necessarily target the most prevalent chronic illnesses, which is where the greatest potential savings lie. To take two examples: (1) HIV ranks #1 in public-health spending, but ranks seventy-fifth on the list of diseases in terms of how many health-care dollars are spent on diagnosing and treating it; and (2) low back and neck pain ranks low in public-health spending, but ranks high in terms of how many health-care dollars are spent on it.*

◊ *Conditions or events that are not necessarily thought of as part of health care are big drivers of health-care spending, including falls, depression, pregnancy, and dental care, all of which were in the top fifteen in terms of health-care dollars spent.*

Perhaps the most provocative item in the above list is that relating to spending on public health and prevention. This is money allocated by the federal government through the National Institutes of Health (NIH) for the purpose of research (R&D) into how best to (a) prevent and (b) treat specific diseases or conditions.

Given a natural public interest in making a major impact on prevention and cure, you'd expect that spending for this purpose would be proportionate to the number of people affected by the disease. Instead — as pointed out by Carolyn Y. Johnson's July 17, 2015, *Washington Post* article "Why the diseases that cause the most harm don't always get the most research money" — the decision to spend more R&D money on one disease and less on another is determined by a complicated combination of considerations, among them: which disease can benefit most from concerted research, that is, may be cured or significantly alleviated; and the severity of the harm suffered by those afflicted with the disease. This last consideration is probably why more public-health attention is not given arthritis, one of the most-common and -painful ailments but not fatal and not always disabling.

The difference in spending increases by disease in the last few years is interesting. An outstanding example is what's been happening with childbirth charges. According to a 2013 study by Truven Health Analytics, the cost of labor and delivery charges has tripled since 1996, and the total cost for pregnancy and newborn care was approximately $30,000 for vaginal delivery in 2013 and $50,000 for a C-section. Some of this may be explained by medical advances that require costlier services, but it's hard not to suspect that there's a certain amount of "what the market will bear" here as well, given the eagerness of most expectant parents.

Public & Private Spending On Which Diseases

The Institute of Health Metrics and Evaluation (IHME) at the University of Washington has released a study of public and private disease-related spending from 1996 through 2013. As the study, published in *JAMA* puts it, "183 sources of data were used to estimate spending for 155 conditions." Here are the numbers for health-care spending in the U.S. by aggregated condition category for 2013:

◊ *$231.1 billion - Cardiovascular diseases*

◊ *$224.5 billion - Diabetes, urogenital, blood, and endocrine diseases*

◊ *$191.7 billion - Other noncommunicable diseases*

◊ *$187.8 billion - Mental and substance-abuse disorders*

◊ *$183.5 billion - Musculoskeletal disorders*

◊ *$168.0 billion - Injuries*

◊ *$164.9 billion - Communicable, maternal, neonatal, and nutritional disorders*

◊ *$155.5 billion - Wellness care*

◊ *$140.8 billion - Treatment of risk factors, e.g. blood pressure,*

◊ *$132.1 billion - Chronic respiratory diseases*

◊ *$115.4 billion - Neoplasms*

◊ *$101.3 billion - Neurological disorders*

◊   *$99.4 billion - Digestive diseases*

◊   *$4.2 billion -   Cirrhosis*

A major purpose of the study was to track increases in spending for categories of disease. There, again, the results were interesting. To use the wording of the study, here is the "annualized rate of change, 1996-2013, in %" — that is, the percentage of increase, year by year in that seventeen-year period, for different categories, as follows:

◊   *6.6% increase - Treatment of risk factors, , e.g. weight, unsafe sex, high blood pressure, tobacco and alcohol consumption, and unsafe water, sanitation and hygiene*

◊   *5.4% increase - Musculoskeletal disorders*

◊   *5.1% increase - Cirrhosis*

◊   *5 .1% increase - Diabetes, urogenital, blood, and endocrine diseases*

◊   *4.0% increase - Neurological disorders*

◊   *3.7% increase - Chronic respiratory diseases*

◊   *3.7% increase - Communicable, maternal, neonatal, and nutritional disorders*

◊   *3.7% increase - Mental and substance-abuse disorders*

◊   *3.3% increase - Injuries*

◊   *3.1% increase - Other noncommunicable diseases*

◊   *2.9% increase - Digestive diseases*

◊   *2.9% increase - Well care*

◊   *2.5% increase - Neoplasms*

◊   *1.2% increase - Cardiovascular diseases*

The One Certainty

In the years ahead all payers — insurance plans, Medicare and Medicaid, individual patients — will resist higher costs and will require greater evidence of total costs and outcomes before approving a course of treatment.

Chapter Five.

Why Health Care Costs So Much In The U.S.

The explanation depends on who's asked. One end of the political spectrum would say that it's because of excessive government participation and regulation, taxes, and unreasonable consumer demands on the system. The other end of the spectrum would say it's because of corporate determination to maximize profits, medical-industry lobbying to maintain special treatment, and a payer system that guarantees reward for inefficiencies. Somewhere in the middle are experts who say it's the expensive, cutting-edge technologies that Americans demand, regardless of expense.

The truth of health-care costs contains elements of all of the above, as well as bottom-line considerations that affect all industries. When considering costs, it's important to remember that health care, in addition to elements specific to its environment, is subject to the same expense pressures as are other industries.

In this chapter, we'll look at several factors with a major impact on costs or that are an issue because of costs, as follows:

◊   *General drivers of costs*

◊   *Specific drivers of health-care costs*

◊   *The role of fragmentation in health-care costs*

◊   *The most-surprising driver of health-care costs*

◊   *The result of increases in health-care costs*

◊   *Health-care rationing*

◊   *What about the cost of health insurance?*

◊   *How health-insurer consolidation affects provider charges*

◊   *How provider size affects costs*

Finally, we'll look at the bottom line on health-care costs, the combination of realities that essentially guarantees that costs will remain high.

General Drivers Of Cost

Costs in any sector of activity are driven by:

◊ *Supply and demand — how many people want the service or product in relation to the amount available*

◊ *Cost of production or provision — what producers and/or providers must pay for labor and materials used in creating and delivering the product or service*

◊ *Overhead — structural expenses that must be built into the end price, such as rent, salaries paid support personnel, accounting expenses, cost of advertising and marketing, interest, legal fees, office supplies and equipment, taxes, travel, utilities, and the like*

◊ *Basic profit requirements — minimum the owners of the business will accept as return on their investment*

◊ *What the market will bear beyond the basic supply-demand equation*

In American health care, each of these general drivers plays a role in pushing costs upward.

Specific Drivers Of Health-Care Costs

Here's a quick overview of the most-significant drivers specific to health care.

◊ *The number of baby boomers entering the phase of their lives when they are more likely to need medical care will keep demand strong. Also, new diagnostic and treatment capabilities will bring more consumers into the system, as will the increase in the number of consumers with health insurance.*

◊ *According to The Commonwealth Fund, health-care spending in the U.S. is much higher than that of other high-income countries, largely because, when compared to other developed nations, prices are higher in the U.S. for identical procedures and also because we're greater users of expensive technologies.*

◊ *The personnel required to provide medical services are, by and large, highly trained and credentialed, and in many occupations, even as demand increases, already in short supply, which will tend to keep salaries higher and benefits more extensive. Also, in health care, as across all industries, the salary expectations of the "people at the top" have escalated. All this translates into ever-higher labor costs.*

◊   *The facilities in which medical services are provided are highly specialized and full of expensive equipment that sometimes has a relatively short life over which its original cost must be amortized.*

◊   *Medical advances require retraining and, often, reequipping. This adds more to the cost of labor and facilities.*

◊   *Medical facilities and practices spend increasing amounts on advertising and marketing-related activities.*

◊   *Patients and providers exposed to marketing and advertising of drugs and other medical products are more likely to seek out products because they are new, and new products are usually more expensive.*

◊   *Patients who research conditions and diseases on the Internet — which increasing numbers are doing — are more likely to seek out and demand treatments that turn out to be unnecessary or even harmful, leading to the purchase of otherwise-unneeded medical services.*

◊   *Some vendors of expensive medical services play games with the 2010 Patient Protection and Affordable Care Act (ACA - Popular Nickname: Obamacare), using convoluted schemes to encourage patients to switch from Medicaid to private insurance which will pay up to four times as much for treatments. In the case of dialysis clinics, for example, this could mean as much as an additional $200,000 per patient per year for the same course of treatment.*

◊   *Government requirements that all parts of the medical industry shift to electronic health records (EHRs) and ICD-10 coding has upped the cost of doing business, especially for small physician practices that find themselves faced with unprecedented IT demands. Ultimately, the IT changes should prove an advantage for both providers and patients, but at the outset their implementation is not only expensive but also tends to slow down operations, which adds to costs.*

◊   *Big Pharma keeps drug prices high by, in effect, extending patent protection. Pharmaceutical companies do this by slightly refining the formulas of older, widely used drugs about to go out of patent protection and so about to lose much of their market value. Their owners then patent the refined variation, price it higher than the original drug, and market it aggressively to physicians as an "improved" version that will be better for their patients. Perhaps the most egregious example of this is the tenfold and more price increase for widely marketed varieties of insulin, which is critical for the treatment of diabetes. Doing this is legal and a legitimate part of a business model, but it definitely adds to costs.*

◊ *The cost of ambulance service has increased due to growth in and consolidation of the for-profit segment of the business.*

◊ *The expectations of investors in the "for profit" part of the medical industry have increased, pressuring managements to squeeze more profits from every activity.*

◊ *Fraud continues to increase to a level that's estimated to be anywhere from 3% to 10% of the total amount spent on health care in the U.S. Health-care fraud is facilitated by: (1) the many different ways in which fraud can be committed; (2) the number of medical-industry participants with an incentive to commit fraud; (3) the efforts of organized crime to perpetrate health-care fraud; (4) the multiplicity of payers; (5) the difficulty of creating software algorithms capable of detecting fraud when claims are submitted; (6) "Prompt pay" legislation requiring that payers pay or dispute claims within thirty days; and (7) the inadequate number of fraud investigators at both state and federal levels. It is difficult for the patient to spot fraud and notify payers because of the sometimes bizarre way in which bills are itemized, submitted, and paid, at least according to the statements seen by the patient. It's evidently difficult even for Medicare to spot fraud — a whistleblower has asserted that insurance companies routinely cheat the government program by "goosing" codes to make Medicare Advantage members appear sicker than they are, which leads to higher government subsidies for the companies. Also playing a role is a sense - widespread until recently — that white-collar crimes like this somehow aren't really serious, even though they threaten the medical system and so affect many more people than the solitary robber taking a wallet at gunpoint.*

◊ *Big Pharma has become increasingly sophisticated in the pricing of new drugs, basing prices not so much on what it costs to develop, manufacture, and market the drug as on how much the drug helps those who will take it and on how much the untreated condition will ultimately cost the health-care system, insurance carriers, and the patient. This inevitably leads to higher prices than when the drug is priced primarily according to actual expenses. For example, as this is* being written, the Food and Drug Administration (FDA) has approved *Spinraza*, the first drug to treat patients with spinal muscular atrophy, which causes muscle damage and weakness that worsens over time and eventually leads to death. About one in ten thousand babies, or four hundred a year in the U.S., are born with this rare disease, which is genetic in origin and a leading cause of death in infants. Adults can be afflicted with a milder form of the disease. *Spinraza* alleviates symptoms in adults and helps afflicted children reach developmental milestones that would otherwise be beyond them. Ultimate impact on life expectancy is unclear. One dose will cost $125,000, and the first year's dosage will cost $625,000 to $750,000. Annual dosage maintenance in subsequent years will cost about $325,000 per patient. It's anticipated that patients afflicted with spinal muscular atrophy will take *Spinraza* throughout their lives. This is but one of several recent miracle drugs that come with hefty price tags.

◊   In the "what the market will bear" category are several trends in health care that go beyond normal supply and demand. For example, unbundling of medical services on bills invariably adds to costs — this is the practice of breaking every activity and supply involved in one process into many separate billing entries. Instead of billing one total amount for a surgical procedure, for instance, a hospital may bill separately for anesthesia, several individual segments of the surgery itself, operating room, recovery room, and medical supplies; and the bill for each surgeon involved is also broken out into detailed segments. Typically, each billing entry includes at least a minor administrative charge. Another trend that increases costs is decreasing competition in the form of hospital mergers and practice consolidation. Studies published in *JAMA* suggest that, when hospitals or networks buy physician practices, average expenditures per patient rise anywhere from 10.3% to 19.85%, and there is an increase of from 8.3% to 16.1% in charges for office visits.

◊   Perhaps the most newsworthy recent cost drivers in the "what the market will bear" category come from the pharmaceutical industry. Most notable is the ongoing consolidation in the industry that relieves pharmaceutical companies of many competitive pressures. In the last twenty years, sixty pharmaceutical companies dwindled to ten even as drug prices went up. Sometimes this involved one giant pharma buying another, as when #1 Pfizer bought Warner-Lambert in 2000, Pharmacia in 2002, Wyeth in 2009, and Hospira in 2015. Sometimes this has involved a company buying one drug, usually older, as when Turing Pharmaceuticals, *a start-up run by a former hedge-fund manager, bought Daraprim, a 62-year-old drug that is the most effective for malaria and the treatment of toxoplasmosis, a life-threatening parasitic infection. Pre-acquisition by Turing, each Daraprim tablet cost $13.50; afterwards, Turing jumped the price to $750.00 a tablet, an increase of over 5,000%.*

◊　*The most arbitrary and widespread way in which pharmaceutical companies push up costs, of course, is their successful lobbying. In 2003 — under pressure from Big Pharma — Congress passed legislation (which seems to have been written by Big Pharma) that bars Medicare from negotiating with drug makers to get lower prices, leaving the government program a sitting duck for price increases that it is powerless to resist. Lifting that prohibition would be one of the quickest ways to cut health-care costs; but, given the amount of money Big Pharma pours into lobbying (over $20 million in the first quarter of 2014 alone), it's unlikely that Congress will act. The rationale for prioritizing Big Pharma's profit goals is that it needs ever-increasing amounts of money for R&D in order to continue to deliver life-enhancing and -lengthening drugs. This argument would be more convincing if, as reported by Healthcare for America Now, drug companies didn't spend nineteen times more on marketing than on R&D.*

◊　*Another way in which prescription-drug use drives up costs is the tendency of patients to assume that there's "a pill for every ill" and to demand it, together with the tendency of many doctors to give them what they want as long as it won't actively harm them.*

The list of drivers increasing costs could go on and on, but what it comes down to is that, even if the system enjoyed maximum efficiency at every point of delivery, health care is an expensive product being effectively marketed by a sophisticated industry to a public ready to consume it at a time when scarcities are developing. And the medical system is in a period of transition when inefficiencies, fraud, and what might most charitably be termed sharp practice are rampant.

The Role Of Fragmentation In Health-Care Costs

The factor that may in the past have had the greatest impact on the rate of cost increases was the fragmentation in U.S. health care. A patient could be seeing a wide range of physicians for various ailments, some of them prescribing duplicative or even contradictory medications. Duplicative tests could be ordered either because the provider did not know they'd already been done at the request of an earlier doctor or simply to beef up revenues. Treatment was rarely coordinated in order to ensure that one part of the care process supported and reinforced any others in which the patient was involved.

To a great extent this unfortunate situation continues, but it's changing. Payer pressure and legislative requirements that providers keep EHRs accessible to the patient and other providers make it more difficult to justify duplication in treatment of patients or billing to payers. Also, new care-delivery models — like Patient-Centered Medical Homes (PCMHs) and ACOs (Accountable Care Organizations) — (1) reward providers who work together to improve outcomes (which also serves to lower costs) and (2) penalize providers who don't.

Another aspect of U.S. health care with an impact on costs has been the lack of connection between population health management and personal patient care. Costs are lower and outcomes better in industrialized countries that consistently use (1) what's been learned from individual-patient care to enhance understanding of population health and (2) the results from analysis of population health observations in fine-tuning individual diagnosis and treatment. This, too, is changing in that recent legislation and regulation encourage using both kinds of care to coordinate better outcomes for populations that share key characteristics.

In the long run, these and other ongoing changes should result in significant savings for payers, a better diagnostic and treatment process for patients, and improved public health.

The Most-Surprising Driver Of Health-Care Costs

To an objective observer, possibly the most-surprising driver of health-care costs is the traditional failure of payers to demand accountability for outcomes. This has two aspects, one that relates to the failure of providers to deliver what they have been paid for and the other that involves patients who do not follow doctor's orders or otherwise undermine the effectiveness of care paid for by their insurance company or employer.

Both forms of unaccountability can produce bizarre situations that are unlike in various ways but that share one outstanding characteristic: they cost a lot of money that produces little that is positive.

To take just one example, in even the very recent past, hospitals that made an error in patient treatment — operated on the wrong location, performed the wrong surgery, allowed a patient to contract an infection that required months of ongoing care, administered the wrong medication that almost killed a patient and required emergency action, etc., etc., etc. — often charged not only for the patient's original contact with the hospital but also for corrective procedures that were necessitated by hospital error. The payers involved usually paid, in effect rewarding the hospitals for having made mistakes. An example of this with which I'm personally familiar is the first, uncompleted stent procedure my husband Robert endured in 2007. The regional medical facility that could not complete the procedure due to its inadequate supply cupboard charged – and was evidently paid by our insurance carriers – almost as much as the facility that subsequently inserted the stents.

As for patients who undermine their medical care, I can recall several acquaintances who never completed physical therapy following orthopedic surgeries. They continued to have problems with what should have been remedied by the original procedures, problems that were addressed through ongoing medical treatment paid for by the same insurance plans that had paid for the original surgery. I have known at least two COPD victims who sneaked cigarettes in between breathing treatments. A young man, a former neighbor, continues to have knee problems for which he regularly seeks treatment. He's been told by several orthopedists that the knee pain is caused by his excessive weight, not surprising given that he's about 5'6" and weighs probably 250 pounds. He angrily rejects this diagnosis and simply goes to another specialist who puts him through the same tests to come up with the same diagnosis, at which point he leaves again for what he thinks will be a more-sympathetic practitioner. He doesn't want to do what it would take to lose the weight, and he thinks he's being cheated when the orthopedist is unable to keep him on a pill that will allow his knees to remain pain-free while his weight continues to balloon.

As long as insurance companies, Medicare and Medicaid, and employers continue to subsidize unaccountability on the part of providers and patients, there is probably little hope for serious cost containment.

The Result Of Increases In Health-Care Costs

Health-care costs significantly exceed the rise in the general cost of living in the U.S. Our costs also compare unfavorably with the cost of health care internationally. A July 2016 Investopedia.com article by Aaron Hankin – "U.S. Healthcare Costs Compared to Other Countries" – analyzed the 2015 *Comparative Price Report* issued by the International Federation of Health Plans (IFHP) and concluded that "not only were U.S. health-care costs elevated compared to the other countries in the survey [the United Kingdom, Switzerland, Australia, New Zealand, South Africa, and Spain], but there is also a marked difference in what people [in different parts of the U.S.] pay... for the same drug or medical procedure."

It should be noted that, as costs increase, so does the percentage of out-of-pocket cost that individual patients pay, even those individuals who are insured. This is because of increases in deductibles and co-pays. As for any attempt to relate individual medical bills to these massive totals, good luck. As mentioned earlier, the way in which patient bills are itemized and coded makes it almost impossible for the uninitiated (and sometimes, I'm told, even the initiated) to get any real sense of what costs how much and how often.

Health-Care Rationing

Before visions of the dreaded "death panels" come to mind, let's agree on what, in the real world, health-care rationing means today, who uses it, and how it works:

◊ *What it means: Health-care rationing is a way to save money and also to spare patients from being subjected to treatments with little chance of success.*

◊ *Who uses it: Payers — including health insurers, government programs, and individual patients.*

◊ *How it works: Treatments are not automatically given patients because they are available, but must have a track record that justifies likely outcomes in relation to cost. Another way it works: Patients are limited by insurer narrow networks as to which providers they can use.*

The last-mentioned form of rationing involves health-insurer networks that limit the doctors the patient can choose, typically doctors with whom the insurance company has negotiated fees in advance. Patients who go "out of network" must usually pay more or all of the resulting bill. Underpinning such financial forms of health-care rationing are purely monetary stipulations written into insurance policies that require co-pays, deductibles, and caps (most are illegal now, but some are still grandfathered), the insurer reasoning being that patients are less likely to overuse health-care resources when they know they must pay some part of the bill and that, ultimately, the insurer will stop payments altogether once a certain limit is reached.

Another form of rationing is denial of care. There are various reasons for denial, but oftentimes it's based on guidelines relating to (1) the medical necessity of treatment, (2) the experimental nature of treatment, (3) potential danger to the patient posed by the treatment, and (4) failure of the treatment to be included in "standards of care" accepted by a professional association or government agency.

A typical rationale for denying treatment is evidence that a treatment either hasn't been proven or has been proven not to work well enough, if at all. Let's say that a new treatment for a particular disease is known to benefit only one of every five hundred patients but costs tens of thousands of dollars. In such a case, whichever payer is going to foot that bill is going to scrutinize very carefully whether or not the cost is disproportionate in relation to the poor statistical outcome. In all likelihood, the uninsured patient who is paying his or her own bills will decide the odds aren't good enough to justify going into debt. As for health insurers and the government, these payers are not going to give automatic approval for unproven treatments and may ultimately reject them and any claims related to them that were not pre-authorized.

Alternative treatments that haven't been tested are another target of rationing, with insurers claiming they can't reimburse for unproven therapies. The insurer isn't saying the patient can't have the treatment, just that the company isn't justified in paying for it due to the ambiguity of outcome or likelihood of failure.

Insurance companies ration health care primarily to (1) control costs and keep premiums lower and therefore more competitive, (2) increase profits, and (3) encourage patients to seek treatments that offer the highest chance of successful outcomes, which tends not only to resolve the immediate issue but also to improve patient health in the long term, thus continuing to lower insurer expenses. Government programs like Medicare ration for purposes of both quality and money. They thereby encourage better outcomes, keep taxes lower, and/or protect the program's ability to expand care that is likelier to achieve a better result for larger numbers of patients.

Even individuals with insurance that will cover a claim sometimes self-ration by choosing to treat themselves — as when they go to the pharmacy for bandages and nonproprietary medicine to treat a bad cut rather than go to an urgent-care center or emergency room, wait to be seen, then go to the pharmacy to get whatever medicine has been prescribed, paying any co-pays and deductibles along the way.

As for the "death panels," the term as originally applied several years ago in somewhat hysterical political propagandizing is misleading. The controversy arose when Medicare-related health-care legislation was about to address the issue of reimbursing physicians for holding end-of-life counseling sessions. The purpose of such sessions was to present patients and their families with options for treatment during the final phases of illness. The goal was to give those concerned more of a voice in how they wish ongoing medical treatment to be handled.

Some physicians and hospitals have been doing this for years. When my widowed mother-in-law June was diagnosed with pancreatic cancer, for example, her doctor discussed with her and her only child, my husband Robert, the treatment options, which were limited. June's doctor shared his experience in assessing what each involved and the degree to which treatment might extend her life. Finally, he mentioned hospice care and explained its nature. He was particularly careful to warn June that, should she choose the hospice option, there would be no more treatment as such but merely the alleviation of pain and discomfort. The doctor answered June and Robert's questions as to the treatments and hospice, but made no particular effort to persuade her to choose one option over another. At his mother's request, Robert sought second and third opinions from specialists and learned that the available treatments were uncomfortable and, in June's case, unlikely to lead to more than a few weeks' prolongation of life. June was a smart, no-nonsense woman in full possession of her mental faculties who had asked the doctors to tell her the truth and was fully capable of making up her mind as to what she wanted to do. She chose hospice. She explained to me that she did this because of the inevitably fatal nature of her illness at the time.

Treatment might — or might not — extend her life a few months even as it subjected her to ongoing discomfort, whereas hospice offered her the opportunity to be pain-free for however much time she had left. She lived another five months, mentally alert and relatively comfortable until days before her death, using the time to enjoy her family and friends. She might have chosen a different route had her disease not been recognized as so quickly terminal, but the point is that the doctors' candor allowed her to choose.

A byproduct, of course, is that her choice saved Medicare and her supplemental insurance carrier money. There are those who seem to feel there is something wrong with patients being told their options if one of the options benefits payers. June would disagree. She viewed honest information as a great blessing.

Anyone who's watched friends or loved ones go through the nightmare of intensive medical care in a hopeless situation, often when they aren't able to protest, understands the need for end-of-life counseling. In the best of all worlds, of course, patients will have completed living wills in which they indicate their preferences in advance as to medical care and name a health-care executor. Unfortunately, as recently as March 2016, according to the American College of Emergency Physicians (ACEP), nearly two-thirds of Americans don't have living wills. Why don't they? The *American Journal of Preventive Medicine* says lack of awareness is the top reason. This suggests that, at the least, end-of-life counseling sessions might encourage patients to draw up such documents so that they can be sure the treatment they get is the treatment they want. Otherwise, they will get whatever treatment is available because that is what providers are set up and — in some circumstances — legally obligated to give them.

In January 2016, Medicare — following recommendations from the AMA — began reimbursing doctors for advance-care planning discussions that address with patients their preferences as to treatment options in the final years and months of life. Previously, this kind of doctor visit had not been billable as a separate service, and many doctors, caught in the pressure to deliver only billable services, had not addressed the issue specifically with patients. The amount that is now paid for such doctor-patient meetings is small, but it's hoped that any payment will increase the frequency of advance planning.

It is logical that Medicare lead the way in this regard because, according to the Henry J. Kaiser Family Foundation, about 80% of the 2.6 million people who died in the U.S. in 2014 were on Medicare. Giving weight to the need for end-of-life planning is the fact that most Americans experience a medically intensive final year in spite of surveys and anecdotal evidence indicating that for decades those contemplating terminal disease have said they prefer to die at home and without extraordinary measures taken to prolong life. An extensive study of Medicare recipients in the 1990s indicated that medical expenditures in the last year of life were five times greater than in non-terminal years; and a more-recent study indicates that the 6% or so of Medicare recipients who die each year account for 27% to 30% of Medicare costs. The numbers are impressive but also discouraging given that they incorporate treatment choices many patients themselves would evidently not have made had they been able.

What About The Cost Of Health Insurance?

And we mustn't forget the cost of health insurance, a medically related expense not included in any of the above figures. Not only has its cost skyrocketed in the last few years, but it will almost certainly continue to rise disproportionately because of consolidation in the industry.

Two recent merger attempts — Anthem Inc.'s $48-billion would-be purchase of Cigna Corp and Aetna Inc.'s $34-billion bid for Humana, Inc. — have lost the first rounds for approval in federal courts. If the cases are appealed and succeed, most analysts assume that disproportionate premium increases will follow the consolidations, which means that both individual policies and employer group policies would cost more, probably leading some employers to require employees to pay a greater share of premium cost.

According to industry insiders, consolidation isn't the only reason for the dramatic rise in insurance costs. J.B. Silvers, professor of health finance at the Weatherhead School of Management at Case Western Reserve University and former health-insurer CEO, says it's also down to the failure of (1) the 2010 ACA to balance incentives so that "too many older, sicker individuals joined, and younger, healthy people were discouraged" and (2) the 2012 (and later) Republican Congress reneging "on its promise to help insurers in the first years of the ACA by limiting risk."

In an Op-Ed piece in *The New York Times* (January 17, 2017), Silvers says:

> *Obamacare, or any plan that replaces it that is reliant on private insurers and individual enrollment, will succeed only under the following conditions: a meaningful incentive to purchase insurance (the individual mandate or equivalent); help to make it more affordable; risk reduction for insurers to stabilize premiums; and enough funding to pay for it all.*

> *If any replacement plan doesn't include these elements, private insurance will revert to the chaos of the pre-A.C.A. market. In business, managing risk is important; in insurance, it is everything. Whoever plays games with it - knowingly or inadvertently - is playing with fire.*

In essence, the name of the game is tradeoffs. If the ACA is repealed in its totality, so that insurers are again allowed to price plans at will for any age group and exclude preexisting conditions, the cost of health insurance may stabilize or even decrease, but millions of people will lose access. If the ACA is repealed in part, so that the mandatory and subsidy elements are eliminated but other provisions are left intact, then it's expected that at least some insurers will exit the market. Insurance is based strictly on numbers related to risk, and the numbers will no longer add up.

How Health-Insurer Consolidation Affects Provider Charges

An interesting byproduct of consolidation is that smaller insurance companies pay more than do larger companies for routine medical services. As this was being written, *Health Affairs* reported that a routine visit to the doctor's office by an insured patient would cost a large insurer $68 and a small insurer $86. This is because the large insurer leverages its size and ability to have a greater overall impact on a provider's income to demand lower rates.

How Provider Size Affects Costs

Just as insurer size affects billing, so does that of providers. The study in *Health Affairs*, cited above, showed that major providers demand higher reimbursements from insurers than do small medical practices. Small practices, for example, billed insurers of medium size an average of $72 for a routine visit, while a large office would bill the same insurer an average of $86. Size clearly matters when it comes to billing, possibly because of services a larger practice is set up to offer. It may also, however, have something to do with a larger practice having the financial buffer to spend longer negotiating billing charges.

The Bottom Line On Health-Care Costs

The bottom line is that in twenty-first-century America costs for all things tend to rise. Costs for a product or service where demand outstrips supply rise more. Costs for an in-demand product or service that can be produced only through a combination of huge amounts of capital and highly trained professionals using expensive facilities rise even more. Health care, together with the insurance industry and government programs that support it, represents a situation in which exponentially increasing costs can be justified by many factors and reined in by few.

The best hope for cost containment involves the new delivery models that now prioritize quality of care over quantity of care, requiring accountability on the part of providers and greater participation of patients. Only when the health-care industry has a serious monetary interest in delivering to patients and payers what actually works will costs begin to stabilize in relation to outcomes.

Chapter Six.

Who Regulates, Influences & Legislates Health Care?

Almost every aspect of health care is controlled by legislation and/or monitored by one regulatory body or another, and sometimes by more than one. The reasons for this complexity are understandable when you think about what's involved.

For starters, life and health are so important that providers of health-related products and services will inevitably become the object of all kinds of government oversight, particularly since, when all programs at all levels are taken into account, government is the largest payer of health-care costs. This leads into the next reason for complexity: turf wars between federal and state authority. Add the "codes of conduct" or "professional standards" to which medical institutions and practitioners subscribe, either individually or through organizations representing their interests, and you've got a lot of paperwork, inspections, and the like.

Here's a brief summary of major regulatory and other health-related players — including corporations, lobbyists, and political contributors — and what in the health-care industry falls primarily or totally into their jurisdictions or within their areas of responsibility or influence.

Local Authorities

Local authorities can control, depending on local statutes, health-industry issues that fall within their territorial jurisdictions, such as:

◊   *Investigation of workplace-related injury or illness*

◊   *Response to workplace violence and criminal behavior directed toward or committed within the health-care environment*

◊   *Issuance of business licenses to health-care providers whose function requires them*

◊   *Inspection of food-preparation premises and certain other* health-industry locations for hygiene and safety

◊   *Inspection of health-care facilities for conformity to fire codes*

◊   *Issuance of building permits for health-care facilities*

The States

The states have control over many aspects of health care, such as:

◊   *Physician licensing*

◊   *Nurse registration*

◊   *Licensing of certain other medical occupations*

◊   *Number of hospital rooms, operating rooms, etc., that can be built*

◊   *State-owned hospital facilities*

◊   *Schools of Medicine in state-owned universities*

◊   *Regulation of health insurance, including all private insurers*

◊   *Authority to set up insurance exchanges to comply with market reforms, such as the 2010 ACA, and also to exercise primary enforcement authority over health-insurance issuers*

◊   *Regulation or oversight of certain aspects of workplace health and safety and investigation of accidents*

◊   *Legislation defining medical liability and medical malpractice — traditionally this is the area in which states have had probably the greatest impact on providers and patients*

◊   *Investigation of criminal activities relating to health care, such as inappropriate behavior by health-care practitioners and insurance fraud*

The Federal Government

The federal government regulates, legislates, and makes policy for many parts of the health-care industry, as follows:

◊   *Food & Drug Administration (FDA) of the U.S. Department of Health and Human Services (DHHS) regulates (among other products) various health-care products, including: drugs — both prescription and non-prescription; biologics — vaccines, blood and blood products, cellular and gene-therapy products, tissue and tissue products; medical devices — all kinds, simple to complex; and dietary supplements.*

◊   *Centers for Medicare & Medicaid Services (CMS) of the DHHS administers Medicare, Medicaid, the Children's Health Insurance Program (CHIP), and the Health Insurance Marketplace. As the largest payer of health-care costs that is also charged with implementing various efficiencies and innovation in the health-care delivery system, CMS strongly influences the entire payer universe through its require-ments as to billing and service-delivery models. CMS's latest major initiative is MACRA (Medicare Access and CHIP Reauthorization Act of 2015), which is the most definitive move thus far toward incentiv-izing physicians for participating in pay-for-performance models and penalizing those physicians who cling to the traditional fee-for-service.*

◊   *Centers for Disease Control and Prevention (CDC) of the DHHS — which describes itself as "the nation's health protection agency" — researches diseases, promotes healthy behaviors and environments, and trains public-health workers. It is in the forefront of tracking disease, especially new viruses, and pinpointing efficient ways to combat spread. The CDC is our primary liaison when international coopera-tion is required to fight the spread of viruses originating elsewhere.*

◊   *National Institute for Occupational Safety and Health (NIOSH), part of the CDC, researches work-related injury and illness and recom-mends methods of prevention.*

◊   *DHHS, its partner agencies, and the states were charged by Title IV of the 2009 American Recovery and Reinvestment Act with improving the nation's health care through health-information tech-nology (HIT) by promoting the meaningful use of electronic health records (EHRs), via incentives and penalties.*

◊   *DHHS enforces the Health Information Privacy provisions of HIPAA (Health Insurance Portability and Accountability Act) - which gives patients rights over their health information and sets rules as to who can have access to health information. DHHS also enforces the Security Rule, a federal law that requires security for health informa-tion held and transmitted in electronic form.*

◊   *Occupational Safety and Health Administration (OSHA) of the U.S. Department of Labor (DOL) sets and enforces workplace standards relating to health and safety and also provides training,* outreach, education, and assistance in relation to these issues. OSHA's jurisdiction includes most private-sector employers and their workers, as well as some public-sector employers and workers.

◊ U.S. Federal Trade Commission (FTC), among its other duties, regulates many types of advertising, including that promoting health-care products or services.

◊ U.S. Federal Bureau of Investigation (FBI), part of the Department of Justice (DOJ), among its other duties, exposes and investigates health-care fraud, with jurisdiction over both federal- and private-insurance programs.

◊ Drug Enforcement Administration (DEA) of the DOJ enforces laws and regulations of the United States pertaining to controlled substances.

◊ Animal and Plant Health Inspection Service (APHIS) of the U.S. Department of Agriculture (USDA), Center for Veterinary Biologics, regulates veterinary vaccines and other types of veterinary biologics.

◊ U.S. Office of Management and Budget (OMB) of the Executive Office of the President produces the President's Budget and mea-sures the quality of government programs, policies, and procedures – including those relating to health care – for compliance with presi-dential policies. OMB also coordinates inter-agency policy initiatives.

◊ U.S. Office of Science and Technology Policy of the Executive Office of the President advises the President on the uses of science and technology to meet U.S. national and international priorities, including those relating to health care. It is particularly concerned with ensuring that Federal investments in science and technology make the maximum contribution to public health, economic prosperity, environ-mental quality, and national security.

◊ U.S. Congressional Budget Office (CBO) of the Legislative Branch generates budget and economic information to Congress to provide a basis for economic and budgetary decisions on federal programs, including those relating to health care.

◊ U.S. Government Accountability Office (GAO) of the Legislative Branch serves as the ultimate audit institution of the federal gov-ernment of the United States through its audits, evaluations, and investigations into how federal money is spent for various purposes by *various governmental departments.*

◊   *U.S. Federal Judiciary of the Judicial Branch rules on various aspects of legislation and also executive acts, including those relating to health care.*

All of the above exert governmental control and/or influence over health-care concerns. Together, they do much to keep health care beneficial to those it's intended to benefit — patients. As to other issues, government regulation works to ensure:

◊   *Ever-improving health outcomes in relation to cost*

◊   *Competency in practitioners who treat us*

◊   *Safety in drugs and health-related products*

◊   *Safety in health-care premises for both patients and employees*

◊   *Truthfulness in the advertising of health products and services*

◊   *Reduction in health-care fraud*

Federal Legislation With Special Significance For Health Care

States legislate on important aspects of health care, particularly those having to do with provider liability, but it is the federal government whose legislation has nationwide impact on all parts of The Provider Universe.

Here are some of the key pieces of federal legislation significantly shaping health care as it is evolving today:

◊   *1965 — The U.S. Congress added Title XVIII to the Social Security Act of 1935, establishing Medicare, and Title XIX, establishing Medicaid.*

◊   *1986 — The Consolidated Omnibus Budget Reconciliation Act (COBRA) gave workers who lose their group health benefits the right to continue those benefits for a period provided they are qualified and pay the entire premium for the continuation of the coverage. It also incorporated the Emergency Treatment and Labor Act (EMTALA), which gives individuals the right to emergency care whether or not they can pay.*

◊   *1996 — The Health Insurance Portability and Accountability Act (HIPAA) gave patients nationwide the right to access their health information and established privacy and security protections for that* information, whether paper or digital in format. It also established protections for employees in relation to group health plans, promoted medical savings accounts, and improved access to long-term care services and coverage. A 2009 CMS final rule issued under HIPAA set the requirement for health-care providers to move to ICD-10 coding for billing.

◊ 2003 – Medicare Prescription Drug, Improvement and Modernization Act added prescription drugs to Medicare and provided more access to comprehensive exams, disease screenings, and other preventive care.

◊ 2009 – Title IV of the American Recovery and Reinvestment Act promoted the "meaningful use" of electronic health records (EHRs) aimed at improving the nation's health care through incentivizing the use of health information technology (HIT) by eligible professionals and hospitals.

◊ 2010 – Patient Protection and Affordable Care Act (ACA - Popular Nickname: Obamacare), among other things, (1) set forth a patient's bill of rights affecting access to health care, (2) provided small business health-insurance tax credits, (3) expanded coverage for key preventive services under Medicare, (4) eliminated the ability of insurance companies to refuse health coverage because of preexisting conditions, (5) limited the degree to which insurance companies could use age as a reason to adjust premiums upward, (6) allowed parents to keep children up to the age of twenty-six insured through their health coverage, (7) lowered costs for drugs in the Medicare "donut hole," (8) empowered CMS to promote and incentivize innovations in care delivery, (9) set up a Prevention and Public Health Fund to invest in proven prevention and public-health programs, (10) cracked down on health-care fraud, and (11) in the 2010 Act's most controversial pro-visions, guaranteed Americans access to affordable health-insurance options through subsidies and other incentives, penalized Americans who did not obtain health insurance, and promoted the expansion of Medicaid.

◊ 2015 – Medicare Access and CHIP Reauthorization Act (MACRA), a bipartisan initiative, introduced the Quality Payment Program (QPP) under which qualifying physicians and other providers (physician assistants, nurse practitioners, clinical nurse specialists, and certified registered nurse anesthetists) must choose to participate *in either a Merit-Based Incentive Payment System (MIPS) or an Accountable Care Organization (ACO) or other Advanced Alternative Payment Model (APM) path. Effective date was January 1, 2017, and participants must submit 2017 performance data by March 31, 2018. Those in MIPS who do not participate at all in 2017 earn a 4% negative adjustment in Medicare payments. MIPS participants who submit data by March 31, 2018, for part of 2017 experience no negative adjustment and may even be eligible for a positive adjustment. MIPS participants who submit data for all of 2017 by March 31, 2018, may be eligible for a larger positive adjustment. Participants via the Advanced APM path may earn a 5% incentive payment in 2019 provided their APM submits data by the deadline. Among the more-significant provisions of MACRA was the requirement that Medicare stop printing Social Security numbers on Medicare cards, thereby addressing a major and longstanding security concern.*

Together, the above are in the process of addressing a wide range of issues relating to the quality and cost of health care. As all are the result of political action — bipartisan or party-specific, theoretically they can be undone by political action. In reality, any changes are likely to address only provisions generally unpopular enough to allow politicians to gain and keep political support for their elimination or significant limitation.

Other Organizations

Other organizations shaping the health-care industry include associations serving providers, such as the AMA, the AHA, Pharmaceutical Research and Manufacturers of America (PhRMA), American Academy of Family Physicians (AAFP), American Nurses Association (ANA), and the like. All such associations have membership standards, and most require adherence to a code of conduct or ethics.

Another influencer is the Liaison Committee on Medical Education (LCME), which provides accreditation of medical-education programs in the U.S. leading to the MD degree.

Also influential are state boards that license physicians and register nurses and private, occupation-specific boards that certify practitioners who voluntarily undergo a stringent examination and vetting process. Board certification is not a legal requirement to practice, but it gives practitioners an edge in an increasingly competitive environment. Also, certification requirements drive ongoing provider interest in the topics tested.

Lobbyists & Political Contributors

Then there's lobbying, not to mention the political contributions that give lobbying much of its clout.

Lobbyists influence (1) legislators who pass bills affecting the interests of the organizations employing the lobbyists and (2) regulators who interpret and enforce legislation, executive orders, and the like. In an era in which issues become ever more complicated, lobbyists can serve a valuable function in making sure that legislators and regulators understand the impact of their actions on the industries represented by the lobbyists.

In 2015, according to the Center for Responsive Politics (whose numbers come from the Senate Office of Public Records), at $509,819,585 spent, health was the second largest lobbying sector, and five of the top fifteen lobbying spenders were in the health-care sector:

◊ *Blue Cross/Blue Shield (#3) - $23,702,049*

◊ *American Medical Association (#4) - $21,930,000*

◊ *American Hospital Association (#7) - $20,687,935*

◊ *Pharmaceutical Research and Manufacturers of America (#9) - $18,920,000*

◊ *CVS Health (#15) - $15,230,000*

Millions more were spent by insurers. America's health-insurance plans, for example, spent $9,590,000 to lobby in 2015.

Generally speaking, the lobbying thrust in the health sector focuses on:

◊ *Increasing federal funding for research or action related to specific diseases, problems, or health trends — such as efforts to combat diabetes, excessive drinking, or obesity*

◊ *Fighting Medicare and Medicaid efforts to save money through initiatives unpopular with providers — such as reductions in fees, move from fee-for-service to pay-for-performance, and move to bundled billing*

◊ *Resisting requirements imposed on health-care providers that the sector feels represent an "undue burden" — such as the switch from ICD-9 to ICD-10, the rate and method of transition to EHRs, and the attempt to require providers to aid in the detection of health-care fraud*

Most lobbying of the federal government is done by consultants working in the Washington, D.C. area, and an interesting statistic is the large number of "revolvers" among these lobbyists. These are lobbyists who have previously been employed by the federal government, usually for the department they now lobby most frequently. Of those retained to lobby for the health sector in 2015, for example, 48.6% were revolvers.

Three of the biggest health-sector lobbying organizations were also major political contributors. In 2014, the last political cycle for which information was available as this was being written, here are the political-contribution numbers:

◊ *Blue Cross/Blue Shield - $4,303,099*

◊ *American Medical Association - $2,067,441*

◊ *American Hospital Association - $2,047,100*

The degree of correlation between lobbying efforts, political contributions, and legislation or regulation specifically benefiting major lobbying organizations is difficult to quantify, and much health-sector lobbying benefits the public interest. At the same time, money tends to exert undue influence when it's spent in these amounts, and you'll notice there are no groups among the top spenders whose specific role is to protect patients or their interests.

Sponsors Of Drug & Product Tests

We've all seen the headlines on our Internet news feed - "New Study Shows X-Product Actually Good For You," with "X-Product" quite often being something that every other medical test ever conducted shows is *not* good for you. In a thoughtful mood, we may ask ourselves how this one test managed to get that result. Typically, however, especially if a prestigious university or hospital is involved and/or we happen to like eating or using it, we're often more inclined to use that headline as an excuse to put "X-Product" back on the shopping list.

Tests can both clarify and confuse health issues. To see why, it's helpful to look at why tests are conducted, by whom, and how.

As to why, according to federal regulation, drugs and devices must be stringently tested before they can be legally sold in the U.S. This is a matter of consumer safety. As patients, we must have absolute confidence in the contents of the prescription bottles we so trustingly turn to throughout our lives. These tests are supposed to be structured by the makers of the drug to answer two basic questions: (1) effectiveness – does the drug do what the maker claims it does; and (2) safety – does the drug have harmful side effects that outweigh its benefits?

Round one of the tests is laboratory-based and does not involve humans. If round one is satisfactory, indicating that the drug is safe to test on humans, the item is tested in various trials on representative populations. The tests are conducted by giving part of the test population the drug being tested and the other part a placebo that has no physical impact on the human test subject (although it can have a psychological impact that affects how the patient feels and even functions, ergo "the placebo effect").

If the part of the population given the drug being tested shows improvement in comparison with those given the placebo and also if there are no side effects that outweigh the health benefits, the results are submitted to the FDA's Center for Drug Evaluation and Research (CDER). CDER must review all the test evidence and decide if the drug has benefits that outweigh any known risks associated with it. If CDER has questions or concerns, it requests additional information from the sponsor of the test. This can lead to the development of more data by the sponsor, or even to a third round of tests. Because of disasters that can be linked to inadequate testing — like the thalidomide tragedy of the 1960s — CDER policy is to err on the side of caution. This can lead to delays that pharmaceutical companies feel interfere with their business processes. CDER, however, is clear as to its mandate.

Only after CDER approves the drug can it be sold in the U.S. This process makes drugs sold here much safer than they would otherwise be.

Even with this relatively cautious CDER-based testing process, however, there are at least four fairly basic problems:

◊   *The outcome of a study can be influenced by the choices as to the population to be included in the test, as well as by how the selection is made as to those given the placebo and those given the drug.*

◊   *It can be difficult for CDER to determine if the information submitted is credible — in other words, has anything been falsified or even slightly adjusted?*

◊   *Human testing that was once performed in the U.S. is increasingly being outsourced to Third World companies that can more easily and cheaply acquire test subjects, and these subjects do not necessarily have the same characteristics (especially as to environment, nutrition, and general physical condition) as the U.S. patients who will ultimately use the drug, if approved.*

◊   *Recurring underfunding of CDER means that it is at times understaffed, and the approval process can take what the drug industry says is much too long. Extensive delay is used as a reason by drug and device makers to attempt to persuade regulators and legislators to weaken or even eliminate testing requirements.*

Not all studies are the result of legal requirements. Some are done for very different purposes — such as product repositioning and the like — and often involve a different approach. The sponsors are usually trying to prove a new theory or disprove earlier theories, such as:

◊   *The causes of a certain disease have now been shown to (1) include something not previously suspected to be a factor or (2) not include something previously assumed to be a factor.*

◊ *A certain kind of diet can/cannot influence longevity.*

◊ *Certain foods are good/bad for consumer health.*

◊ *Certain herbs and spices can/cannot provide specific health benefits.*

◊ *Certain lifestyle habits can/cannot enhance physical endurance.*

Such studies usually (but not always) involve sizable population samples observed over a period of from months to, more often, years. There are certain protocols generally observed in assembling and monitoring those populations, but not always. There is, in other words, more than a little flexibility as to how and with whom studies are performed.

Those conducting the studies are often academics working at prestigious universities whose professional futures are tied to study results. Those sponsoring the studies — which can be very expensive — may be disinterested parties who have a strong motivation to learn the truth, whatever the truth is. They may also, however, be highly interested parties trying to use the studies "to get their side of the story out." For example, if your industry is based on a product that study after study has found to be generally injurious to health, you'd find it very useful to have a study that appears to prove otherwise. There are several ways for sponsors to influence the impact of studies, directly or indirectly, and the influence doesn't have to be exerted as blatantly as going to a clinician and saying, "Be sure you get this outcome."

Even without undue influence, there seems to be an instinctive bias toward outcomes that in one way or another favor the study's sponsor. A March 2017 interview in *Nutrition Action Health Letter* quotes Marion Nestle, the Paulette Goddard Professor in the Department of Nutrition, Food Studies, and Public Health at New York University, as saying, "For a year, I collected studies that were funded by the food industry... I found 168 studies and 156 of them had results that were favorable to the sponsor. Only 12 didn't." Clearly, this is a statistically improbable outcome. In Dr. Nestle's opinion, those conducting such studies are unconscious of the sponsor influence.

Whether sponsor-influenced or neutral, such studies can have a powerful impact on consumers who view whatever statement follows "A recent study shows that..." as credible, especially when the announcement is covered in what are considered "news of record" media such as *The New York Times, The Guardian, Washington Post,* and other publications that regularly feature health news. The combination of (1) prestigious institutions, (2) highly credentialed researchers, and (3) respected news outlets almost guarantees credibility.

So, how reliable are tests?

It is troubling that even highly expert insiders have come to question the validity of many tests. Take this quote, for example, from the January 15, 2009, article in *The New York Review of Books* entitled "Drug Companies & Doctors: A Story of Corruption:"

> *It is simply no longer possible to believe much of the clinical research that is published... I take no pleasure in this conclusion, which I reached slowly and reluctantly over my two decades as an editor of The New England Journal of Medicine.*

The author was Marcia Angell, M.D., member of the faculty of Global Health and Social Medicine at Harvard Medical School and former Editor-in-Chief at *The New England Journal of Medicine*, one of the most highly respected medical journals in the world.

It's likely, in fact, that the influence of many studies relates as much to the quality of publicity surrounding them as to their inherent worth.

Chapter Seven.

The Scope & Nature Of American Health Care

Sooner or later, just about all Americans need health care. Unless you're born at home without medical attendance, avoid vaccinations, never have an accident or become ill, and drop dead from a heart attack or are killed instantly in an accident, you will experience at least some health care.

Throughout life, in fact, most Americans consume a lot of health care. In this chapter, we'll look at a few facts that indicate its scope and nature.

Most Common Adult Diseases In The U.S.

In alphabetical order, the most-common adult diseases are:

◊   *Arthritis*

◊   *Cancer*

◊   *Diabetes*

◊   *Heart conditions*

◊   *Obesity*

◊   *Stroke*

In 2012, nearly 117 million adults in the U.S. were affected by one or more of these chronic conditions. Hypertension and high cholesterol — both stroke and heart-disease risk factors — also affect many Americans. In 2014, 83.2% of American adults had contact with a health-care professional.

Most-Common Childhood Ailments In The U.S.

In order of their prevalence, the most-common childhood ailments are:

◊   *Common cold*

◊   *Respiratory syncytial virus (RSV)*

◊   *Roseola*

- ◊ *Gastroenteritis*
- ◊ *Hand-foot-mouth disease*
- ◊ *Bright-red cheek rash*
- ◊ *Strep throat*
- ◊ *Influenza*
- ◊ *Pinkeye*
- ◊ *Pinworms*

In 2014, 92.4% of American children had contact with a health-care professional for one or more of the above ailments.

Americans & Their Doctors

In 2014, there were 928.6 million physician-office visits by Americans. Physicians remain the initial point of contact for most individuals who develop symptoms.

According to ZocDoc.com, the top ten qualities that patients value in a doctor, in order, are:

- ◊ *Professionalism*
- ◊ *Friendliness*
- ◊ *Niceness*
- ◊ *Ability to make patient feel comfortable*
- ◊ *Helpfulness*
- ◊ *Expertise*
- ◊ *Empathy*
- ◊ *Kindness*
- ◊ *Ability and willingness to listen*
- ◊ *Thoroughness*

Americans like their doctors, and doctors need patients to justify their career choice. At the same time, the doctor-patient relationship can be difficult. Doctors who manifest behaviors that a patient doesn't like may not be trusted, and their treatment plans may be ignored.

What Patients Don't Like In A Doctor

Doctor behaviors that patients dislike most include, in order:

◊ *Doesn't listen*

◊ *Spends too little time with the patient*

◊ *Is disrespectful*

◊ *Keeps patient waiting*

◊ *Rations care by refusing to recommend anything not sanctioned by the network(s) to which the doctor belongs*

◊ *Puts the patient's interests last.*

It's interesting to compare the above with patient behaviors that are particularly disliked by doctors.

What Doctors Don't Like In A Patient

Patient behaviors most disliked by doctors include, in order:

◊ *Late for appointments*

◊ *Unrealistic expectations as to personal assistance from doctor's office*

◊ *Failure to take medications and to admit this to the doctor*

◊ *Self-diagnosis*

◊ *Delaying doctor as the appointment ends*

◊ *Expectation that treatment and/or medicine can eliminate the need for lifestyle changes*

◊ *Failure to pay bill or make arrangements for payment in a timely manner*

Discord, voiced and unvoiced, between doctors and patients can make patients resistant to the doctor's recommendations, but this is not the only reason patients sometimes question what their doctor tells them.

Why Patients May Question Doctor Treatment Choices

The most basic reason that patients may question treatment choices is that they don't want to follow the doctor's plan. Perhaps it's different from one that worked for someone they know. Maybe it's alarming in some way. Perhaps the patient simply doesn't like it. There are, however, several other reasons a patient may question the doctor's treatment choices.

◊ *When doctor and patient are of different ethnicities, there may be either a lack of trust or perhaps even an inability to communicate due to language difficulties.*

◊ *Some doctors don't take women's health concerns as seriously as they do those of men. Symptoms that get a man sent for medical testing too often get a woman a prescription for tranquilizers and advice "to just calm down."*

◊ *Some patients don't like doctors of a different sex, particularly if their medical problem involves parts of the body considered private. Their discomfort may make them less likely to accept the doctor's assessment of what's wrong and what needs to be done.*

◊ *Overweight patients say that many doctors find it hard to see beyond their size and tend to attribute medical problems to the weight issue without looking further.*

◊ *Patients don't like for doctors to use threats to try to get them to change lifestyle behaviors, as in "If you don't stop smoking, you'll die sooner" and the like. Instead of viewing this kind of information as helpful, many patients view it as a form of prejudice that colors every-thing the physician does.*

◊ *Patients who dare to question the doctor's diagnosis say that once they ask or say anything that implies disagreement, the doctor tends to either back away or become aggressive.*

◊ *The doctor's failure to like a patient may subliminally influence his or her diagnostic and treatment choices, and patients are better at picking up on a dismissive attitude than most doctors appear to realize.*

◊ *The use of heuristics — rapid diagnosis based on physician expe-rience, sometimes precluding other possibilities — makes some patients think that no careful consideration has been given their condition.*

◊ *Related to the above, many doctors, particularly some specialists, have a "one approach fits all" mindset and recommend the same treat-ment for all patients with similar symptoms without exploring other options.*

Sometimes, physician biases are plain from the start. Whether initially obvious or not, they tend ultimately to reveal themselves, making the patient suspicious. Generally, these suspicions are almost certainly unfounded. It's unlikely that a competent physician will not do everything he or she can to help a patient get better as quickly as possible. Unfounded or not, suspicion of physicians and/or their biases is used by some patients to justify resistance to doctor's orders.

Which Surgeries Are Performed Most Often In The U.S.

Of the 40-50 million surgeries performed annually in the U.S., in order, according to HealthGrades, these are the ten most common:

◊   *Cataract removal*

◊   *C-section for surgical delivery of baby*

◊   *Joint replacement*

◊   *Circumcision*

◊   *Broken bone repair*

◊   *Angioplasty and atherectomy to open coronary arteries clogged with plaque and to remove the plaque*

◊   *Stent procedure to keep artery open following angioplasty*

◊   *Hysterectomy*

◊   *Gallbladder removal*

◊   *Heart-bypass surgery*

Surgery has become both more common and safer than in years past. The reason for the increase is that more procedures are available, as are more outlets in which to have them. The increase in safety relates to the improvement in surgical techniques, highly targeted drug therapies, and the fact that patients, even when their surgery is performed on an inpatient basis, spend less time hospitalized and so are less exposed to hospital-spread superbugs.

Who Goes To The Emergency Room In The U.S. & Why

In 2014, 136.3 million Americans went to hospital emergency rooms. Hospital admission followed for 16.2 million, with 2.1 million going to a critical-care unit.

The four most common complaints in American emergency rooms are: abdominal pain; respiratory infections; sprains and strains; and superficial injury.

It should be mentioned that uninsured patients are more likely to go to the emergency room, whether the condition is an emergency or not, because emergency rooms must provide treatment whether or not the patient can pay. This requirement was set forth in the 1986 Emergency Treatment and Labor Act (EMTALA), passed by Congress as part of COBRA.

Who Goes To The Hospital & Why

In 2014, 7.3% of Americans were hospitalized.

In 2010, the ten most frequent reasons for hospitalization, in order, were:

◊ *Liveborn (newborn infant)*

◊ *Pneumonia*

◊ *Osteoarthritis*

◊ *Congestive heart failure (nonhypertensive)*

◊ *Septicemia*

◊ *Mood disorders*

◊ *Cardiac dysrhythmias*

◊ *Chronic obstructive pulmonary disease and bronchiectasis*

◊ *Complication of device (implant or graft)*

◊ *Obstetrics-related trauma to perineum and vulva*

A couple of decades ago, patients would have been hospitalized for many events that today are treated on an outpatient basis.

Who Goes To Intensive Care Units & Why

A 2013 study by George Washington University School of Public Health and Health Services (SPHHS) found that American ICU admissions jumped from 2.79 million in 2002-2003 to 4.14 million in 2008-2009.

Patients are admitted to the ICU because they need either close monitoring or special treatment in connection with one or more of the following situations:

◊ *After a major surgical operation or serious head injury*

◊ *Problems with lungs that require ventilator support with breathing*

◊ *Heart and blood-vessel problems*

◊ *Chemical imbalance in the bloodstream*

◊ *Serious infection requiring specialized ICU care*

The ICU is not only the scene of the highest mortality rates but also one of the most-expensive medical settings, as well as an environment where medical errors are most likely to occur because of the complexity of care.

Prescription Drug Use & Misuse

A 2013 Mayo Clinic study revealed that 70% of Americans take at least one prescription drug. More than half of Americans take two prescription medications, and 20% take at least five prescription medications.

The most commonly prescribed drugs are antibiotics, antidepressants, and opioids. Other frequently prescribed drugs are vaccines, cholesterol-lowering drugs, and anti-asthma drugs.

Most of the time, prescription drugs are used properly, but not always. Abuse is the misuse of prescription drugs in one of these ways:

◊ *Using a drug that isn't prescribed for the patient and/or the patient's condition*

◊ *Using a drug in the wrong quantities or at the wrong intervals*

◊ *Using a drug simply for the experience of taking the drug, i.e., it provides a high or a feeling of pleasure or some other desired sensation*

Prescription-drug abuse is a serious societal issue because it harms not only abusers but also those with whom they work, live, and share the highway. The most commonly abused medications are:

◊ *Pain relievers*

◊ *Tranquilizers*

◊ *Stimulants*

◊ *Sedatives*

Some abused medications are bought on the street, but others are provided by friends or relatives or are simply removed from family medicine cabinets where they're kept because another occupant of the house has a prescription for the drug.

Certain prescription drugs are abused in such significant numbers that the DEA (Drug Enforcement Administration) aggressively investigates the issue, making some physicians reluctant to prescribe those medications even though seriously ill patients, particularly those suffering from cancer, need them to control excruciating pain.

Physician choice of a specific drug to prescribe can be broad, for many drugs can be used to treat the same conditions. Oftentimes, they are very similar with only minor differences in their composition that do not affect their impact. Sometimes, the differences are great enough to cause different side effects, meaning that a physician may change the prescription to a similar drug should the side effects prove troubling.

Pharmaceutical companies affect drug choices through advertising and marketing directed to either physicians and/or patients and also through direct appeals to physicians.

Leading Causes Of Death In The U.S.

Not every medical intervention is permanently successful, and sometimes there is no opportunity for intervention.

According to the Centers for Disease Control and Prevention (CDC), the leading causes of death in the U.S. in 2015 were:

◊   *Heart disease - 614,348*

◊   *Cancer - 591, 699*

◊   *Chronic lower respiratory diseases - 147,101*

◊   *Accidents (unintentional injuries) - 136,053*

◊   *Stroke (cerebrovascular diseases) - 133,103*

◊   *Alzheimer's disease - 93,541*

◊   *Diabetes - 76,488*

◊   *Influenza and pneumonia - 55,227*

◊   *Nephritis, nephrotic syndrome, and nephrosis - 48,146*

◊   *Intentional self-harm (suicide) - 42,773*

You'll notice that two of the categories — #4 Accidents and #10 Suicide — are not directly due to illness. You'll notice also that "medical error" does not appear on the list — this is because such deaths are often attributed to the underlying condition from which the patient was suffering and not to the error that precipitated death.

Why Americans Are Such Massive Consumers Of Health Care

We use a lot of health care, and the reasons are seemingly contradictory. For starters, many of us subscribe to the "every day in every way I'm getting better and better" school of thought. We feel it is our responsibility, as well as our right, to make ourselves as good as we can be. This makes us more likely to go to the doctor faster than we otherwise would when a symptom develops. Another factor is our obsession with age and physical appearance - we want to look as good as possible as long as possible. Healthier people look better and age better.

In spite of this obsession, however, we enjoy lifestyles that make us less likely to remain healthy. Most Americans are guilty of one or more of the following:

◊   *We eat too much, and by and large our diet is not nutritionally balanced.*

◊   *We get too little exercise.*

◊   *We live stressful lifestyles.*

◊   *We participate in risky sexual behaviors.*

◊   *We drink too much.*

◊   *We smoke too much.*

◊   *We abuse drugs, recreational and/or prescription.*

◊   *We're not careful about exposure to germs.*

◊   *We're careless in our use of toxic products, like household cleaners.*

Facilitating our use of health care is that — in spite of its problems — by and large we have an excellent health-care system with many specialists to address almost every problem.

In essence, Americans are good consumers of health care because (1) we perceive its benefits, (2) our habits make it necessary, and (3) it's available.

Chapter Eight.

Medical Advances, Medical Miracles

To a great extent, "miraculous medicine" is either here or visible on the near horizon. It's been estimated that the medical knowledge base has been doubling every five to eight years, further that the pace of this doubling is accelerating. (Boston Commons High Tech Network estimates that, "by 2020, medical knowledge doubling time is projected to be 73 days.") The resulting medical advances in diagnosis, treatment, devices, surgical techniques, and pharmaceuticals offer incredible opportunities for patient care. The most-prominent element in medical advances is the increasing personalization of medicine, made possible by testing and treatments derived from the genetics/genomics approach to health care. Tests once told simply what was wrong with a patient. These more-sophisticated tests are so precise that their results can be used to create therapies targeted specifically to an individual patient. This is known as precision medicine, and it will ultimately shape all approaches to health care in The Provider Universe.

Meanwhile, what follows represents just a few of our currently delivered medical miracles.

- ◊ *Dramatic diagnostics*

- ◊ *Target-hitting pharmaceuticals*

- ◊ *New joints for old bones*

- ◊ *Robotic exoskeletons*

- ◊ *Bone marrow/blood stem-cell transplants*

- ◊ *Organ transplants*

- ◊ *Evolving surgical devices and techniques*

- ◊ *Outpatient cataract surgery*

Finally, we'll take a look at the significance of medical miracles for patients and the characteristics that all such miracles share.

Dramatic Diagnostics

Some of the most-dramatic advances have been made in diagnostics. A few years ago, for example, x-rays provided the only way doctors could "see inside" the patient's body, which was good for revealing bone structure, the size and location of tumors, an enlarged heart, blocked blood vessels, and certain digestive-tract problems. Today, x-rays are still used, but CT (computed tomography) scans give greater detail, revealing more about muscle and bone issues, tumor or blood-clot location, internal bleeding or infection, and the like. MRI (magnetic resonance imaging) scans, while not as good as x-rays or CT scans for showing details of bony structures, provide greater detail about soft tissue, detail that is especially useful in examining brain tumors, ligament and tendon injuries, etc.

The number of blood tests has exploded in recent decades, each offering information about the patient in relation to one or more diseases or conditions. This enables doctors to pinpoint much more precisely what is wrong with the patient, which in turn suggests how to deal with it. According to the National Heart, Lung, and Blood Institute (NHLBI), the most-common blood tests are: a complete blood count; blood chemistry tests; blood enzyme tests; and blood tests to assess heart-disease risk. Common or uncommon, blood tests can help to confirm a condition early enough for more-effective intervention.

Common urine tests include urinalysis (UA), urine culture, and urine electrolyte levels. One of the most useful tests is the rapid urine test which involves dipping a test strip in urine to detect pH value, protein, sugar, nitrite, ketone, bilirubin, red blood cells, and white blood cells.

One of the newest diagnostic tools is Face2Gene, a medical app that can — using millions of tiny calculations in rapid succession — analyze facial characteristics in a photo to quantify, compute, and rank them, as Megan Molteni puts it in a January 9, 2017, article in WIRED, "to suggest the most probable syndromes [illness or group or symptoms] associated with the facial phenotype. There's even a heat map overlay on the photo that shows which of the features are the most indicative match."

These and other advances in diagnosis are not only capable of spotting problems earlier, but also make it easier for doctors to determine pharmaceutical and/or surgical approaches and more-effective maintenance regimens for chronic illness.

Target-Hitting Pharmaceuticals

Highly targeted drugs control a wider range of diseases once quickly fatal or disabling. For example, leukemia — a diagnosis that just a few years ago likely meant an imminent death sentence — can now be managed indefinitely with chemotherapy drugs, corticosteroids, monoclonal antibodies, and/or tyrosine kinase inhibitors, depending on the type of leukemia. According to the Leukemia & Lymphoma Society (LLS), the five-year relative survival rate for this disease has more than quadrupled since 1960, more than doubled since the mid-1970s.

One of the most-spectacular target-hitting pharmaceutical therapies is immunotherapy, which uses drugs to target the body's immune system so that white blood cells (T cells) are stimulated to attack diseased cells. Immunotherapy, which treats multiple types of cancer, is superior to conventional cancer therapy that treats only a specific type. Thus far, it's working best on melanoma, non-small cell lung cancer, bladder cancer, and lymphoma. Immunotherapy has generated a lot of excitement in the medical world, but experience revealed that "checkpoints" developed that prevented the therapy from working after a certain point. This has shifted the focus to developing immunotherapy drugs that don't "turn off." As Padmanee Sharma, M.D., Ph.D., physician and researcher, put it in a June 1, 2016, interview published on the MD Anderson Cancer website, "When people talk about immunotherapy right now, they're usually talking about immune checkpoint therapy." Dr. Sharma is confident that the obstacles will be overcome and says that "In 10 years, I think immunotherapy will be the backbone of a lot of our cancer treatments."

Landscape-changing drugs are ever on the horizon. As this book is being written, an article in the *New England Journal of Medicine* reveals trials on Ocrelizumab, a drug that has the potential to slow damage to the brain for multiple sclerosis (MS) sufferers. The drug, described as a landmark in treating MS, depletes B cells to stop their being used by the illness to further damage the body. At almost the same time, an article in *The New York Times* announced that a "100%-effective" Ebola vaccine has been developed and stockpiled, even while extensive testing continues.

Another form of target-hitting has to do with timing. Drugs taken orally normally last no more than a day, and the development of longer-lasting oral medication has been a goal for many researchers. In November 2016, it was announced that a pill has been developed that releases its medicine for two weeks after being swallowed. The revolutionary pill requires further testing, but — once fine-tuned and approved — it's capable of being a game-changer in drug therapy, especially for patients like children or mentally challenged adults who may not always remember to take medication on a daily schedule.

It's anticipated that, ultimately, genetics/genomics will make possible drugs almost certain to work because they're designed specifically for one individual.

Bone-Marrow/Blood Stem-Cell Transplants

The first successful human bone-marrow transplant occurred in 1968, and the use of this treatment — especially for certain types of cancer — has grown significantly. The most-abundant supply of stem cells for transplants comes from bone marrow provided by the patient or a compatible donor, but stem cells can also be collected from the bloodstream or an umbilical cord. According to the Blood & Marrow Transplant Information Network (InfoNet), more than 100 diseases — most commonly blood cancers, certain autoimmune diseases, and tumors — can potentially be treated with blood stem-cell transplants, often with dramatic results.

Organ Transplants

Today, transplantation requires removing healthy organs from donors to replace diseased or injured organs in compatible recipients. According to the United Network for Organ Sharing (UNOS), seven types of organ transplants are now performed in the U.S., including: kidney; pancreas; liver; heart; lung; intestines; and vascularized composite allografts (VCAs) like face and hand transplantation. Kidney transplants are the most common, intestines the least. Double transplants can be done — heart/lung, for example.

Transplantation is dangerous and difficult. There's a risk of infection. There may be highly unpleasant side effects. The organ may be rejected. Wait times for a compatible organ can be agonizing. Also, transplantation is extremely expensive.

Recipients choose to take the risk because their condition is terminal. Most recipients are below the age of sixty. The American Transplant Foundation (ATF) says that there have been over 650,000 transplants in the U.S. since 1988, most of which served to extend patient life span and/or improve quality of life for patients.

New Joints For Old Bones

Joint replacement can significantly improve quality of life by reducing pain and improving mobility. The technique has been around for a long time, but today's joint replacement — especially of large joints like hips and knees — makes use of personalized implants and procedures to give patients shorter hospital stays, quicker recovery, reduced physical-therapy times, and enhanced mobility. The use of plastic in joint implants promises to add to their longevity.

Robotic Exoskeletons

In nature, exoskeletons are a hard outer shell with joints, an external structure capable of supporting and protecting an animal's body (crabs, for example, have exoskeletons).

Robotic exoskeletons not only help human beings move around in difficult conditions and lift weights otherwise beyond their strength, but also make it possible for paralyzed people to walk again. Powered exoskeletons can be used to get victims of stroke, brain injury, and spinal-cord injury back on their feet and functioning.

Evolving Surgical Devices & Techniques

The nature and quality of surgical devices improves continually. To take a recent example, the use of stents in opening clogged arteries has been a lifesaver for many victims of heart disease. The first stents were bare metal, then came drug-eluting stents, both of which remain in place, keeping arteries open. In July 2016, the FDA approved Abbott Laboratories' dissolving stent, already in use in over 100 countries, which after it dissolves leaves behind nothing but a functioning, restored blood vessel. This last has a special interest for me because Dr. Charles "Chuck" Simonton, Abbott's Divisional Vice President, Medical Affairs and Chief Medical Officer/Vascular, is the physician who — in one of his last two months as a practicing surgeon before joining Abbott in December 2007 — performed my husband Robert's three-stent insertion. The dissolving stent made Abbott #5 on *Fast Company's* March 2017 list of the ten most innovative companies in the biotech sector.

And if dissolving stents aren't miraculous enough, how about robot surgeons? The 2016 Nobel Prize in chemistry was awarded for the design and synthesis of the world's smallest machines, nanoscale, i.e., 1,000 times smaller than the width of a human hair. The long-time dream is that they can ultimately be used in nanorobotic surgery and localized drug delivery. In synthetic biology, this could even lead to the development of an artificial cell that can self-divide.

Outpatient Cataract Surgery

We'll end this abbreviated glimpse at a handful of the most-significant medical advances already in place with cataract surgery. There is no treatment for cataracts other than surgical removal. Prior to the late 1980s, this was serious business, requiring what amounted more or less to a dissection of the eye and several days in the hospital as for any major surgery. Today's laser cataract surgery is typically performed on an outpatient basis, is faster and safer, and produces a consistently higher-quality outcome.

Fast Company's 2017 List Of The Ten Most-Innovative Companies In The Biotech Sector

It's interesting to see what *Fast Company's* annual Most Innovative Companies issue honors in what the forward-looking publication describes as "the 10 most exciting companies across the world's most vibrant industries."

The biotech-sector list includes "old line" companies like Johnson & Johnson (founded 1886), Abbott (founded 1888), and Medtronic (founded 1949), as well as relative newcomers like 23andMe (founded 2006) and Celmatix (founded 2009). The list shows that precision medicine is definitely here or in view, for six of the companies were recognized for advancing medicine through their creative use of genetics/genomics and immunotherapy.

How Much Do Medical Miracles Matter?

Thanks to the medical advances of the last few years, individuals who enter the current health-care system are — generally speaking — diagnosed faster and with greater accuracy, treated more efficiently, and sent back to their normal routine in less time with a better outcome.

In the last century, thanks largely to prevention made possible by medical advances, worldwide life expectancy has increased approximately thirty years, from less than forty to approximately seventy. Vaccination is responsible for much of the increase in life expectancy. Some of the once-widespread and often-fatal diseases now capable of being prevented through vaccine include: tetanus; rabies; polio; yellow fever; rinderpest; whooping cough; measles; and smallpox.

More-specific diagnosis and highly targeted interventions, as mentioned above, have made it possible to manage once-fatal diseases like diabetes, leukemia, many other forms of cancer, and heart disease.

The rapidly evolving possibilities of medical care are transforming the quality of life and even extending life spans for millions of Americans who just a few years ago would have died or endured ongoing disability or diminished physical or mental capacity.

All of that has already happened. When you add to the current crop of advances those that are anticipated, perhaps already on the way, we reach a point where, it is predicted, the health-care process may be able to stop and even reverse aging. (Check out **Chapter Thirteen**, *Major Challenge: Medical Advances And New Technology* for more on what's coming.)

What All Medical Miracles Share

All medical miracles — whether one of the few mentioned above or one of the many unmentioned — share commonalities with significant implications for what's going on in American health care today.

◊   *They extend life and/or improve the quality of life for many patients who would otherwise die or live significantly impaired lives.*

◊   *They do not equally benefit all patients with similar problems.*

◊   *They sometimes lead to solutions for issues not necessarily related to the original purpose for which they were developed.*

◊   *They require retraining of practitioners and, sometimes, change in facilities, equipment, or supplies kept on hand.*

◊   *They are expensive.*

Because they require a certain amount of time to "prove themselves" in wide use, are not universally consistent in their effects, and are costly, medical miracles will probably become part of an ongoing and increasingly intense national debate about health-care rationing.

Heavy Hitters In Pursuit Of Medical Miracles

A bright spot in the ever-expanding search for cures and treatments, as well as their implementation, includes privately funded, highly targeted health-related initiatives. Outstanding among current business leaders pursuing this level of philanthropy are billionaires Bill Gates, Warren Buffet, and Mark Zuckerberg, who on *Forbes's* 2017 list of the richest people in the world rank respectively as numbers one, two, and five.

The Bill and Melinda Gates Foundation — with the active support of Warren Buffet — has invested over $36.7 billion in health initiatives, many targeting specific diseases in some of the poorest countries in the world, diseases substantially eradicated or controlled long ago in the developed world.

The Chan Zuckerberg Initiative has announced that it will invest $3 billion dollars over the next ten years to tackle all diseases. The effort will focus on biohub research to bring together scientists and engineers to develop tools to treat diseases, including not only devices but also information, such as what neurobiologist Cornelia Bargmann, leader of the initiative, describes as a "cell atlas" mapping the locations and characteristics of all of the cells in the human body. The output of the initiative will be shared across the scientific community to encourage greater participation in R&D relating to health care.

Today's crop of wealthy people investing in health is not the first, of course. For example, in 1901, John D. Rockefeller, richest man of his day and founder of probably the best-known family dynasty in American history, worked with his son John D., Jr., to found the Rockefeller Institute for Medical Research, the first devoted exclusively to biomedical research. In 1910, this was followed by the Rockefeller University Hospital, the first devoted to clinical research. Involvement with medicine became something of a family tradition. John D., Jr.'s youngest son David, who died at the age of 101 in March 2017, first served on the board of the Rockefeller Institute for Medical Research in 1940 and then in the 1960s helped to transform the Institute into The Rockefeller University, the first U.S. educational institution dedicated to biomedical research. David's son Richard became a Harvard-trained family doctor whose philanthropic causes included the treatment of PTSD (post-traumatic stress syndrome), curing sleeping sickness in Africa, promoting Doctors Without Borders, and widening philanthropic support for the Drugs for Neglected Diseases Initiative (DNDI).

If the descendants of Warren Buffet, Bill and Melinda Gates, and Priscilla Chan and Mark Zuckerberg similarly follow their parents' example, an extremely valuable resource will be continued into the indefinite future, the kind of resource capable of producing startling leaps in health and longevity.

Chapter Nine.

Medical & System Failures

What's happening in health care today seems — and often is — miraculous. There are, however, dark spots in that rosy picture:

◊   *Ways in which we could improve health but don't*

◊   *Diseases that by their nature are difficult to eradicate or cure*

◊   *The rise of antibiotic-resistant bacteria, probably the single most dangerous development in health care today*

Some of these are failures of medical practice and some of will; the last demonstrates the alarming possibility of the impermanence of cures.

Ways In Which We Could Improve Health But Don't

There are many ways in which we could improve health but don't. These failures are caused by personal preferences, employment issues, pollution, lifestyle choices, and public policy. Here are a few examples:

◊   *Vaccine-preventable diseases remain an issue, even in the U.S., mostly because some parents choose, for one reason or another, not to allow vaccination of their children and some adults don't get vaccinations for themselves due to ignorance, indifference, or religious concerns. On the World Health Organization's current list of vaccine-preventable diseases are: anthrax, cholera, dengue fever, diphtheria, haemophilus influenza type b, hepatitis A, hepatitis B, hepatitis E, HPV (human papilloma-virus, influenza, malaria, measles, meningitis (meningococcal disease), mumps, pneumococcal disease, poliomyelitis, rabies, rotavirus gastroenteritis, rubella, shingles (varicella and herpes zoster), smallpox, tetanus, tick-borne encephalitis, tuberculosis, typhoid fever, whooping cough (pertussis), and yellow fever. The results of not getting vaccinated can lead not only to catching the disease but also to serious side effects, like amputation, hearing loss, convulsions, brain damage, disability, disfigurement, and even death.*

◊   *Exposure standards for workers as to toxic chemicals are lower than is known to be safe. Due to successful lobbying efforts by industry, OSHA is not allowed to set exposure standards for employees that conform even to those set by the EPA. Among the diseases or medical conditions that can affect overexposed workers or their children are: allergies, Alzheimer's, asthma, attention deficit disorder, autism, birth defects, cancer, chemical sensitivities, chronic fatigue, depression, diabetes, eczema, heart disease, infertility, inflammatory bowel disease, learning difficulties, multiple sclerosis, Parkinson's disease, reproductive dysfunction, thyroid disease, etc.*

◊   *We allow levels of air pollution that can cause diseases that are mild to severe and include asthma, COPD, lung cancer, mesothelioma, and other breathing-related conditions. (My grandmother, a homemaker in a small town, died of mesothelioma, typically an industrial ailment. The culprit was a small manufacturer a couple of miles upwind who used asbestos.)*

◊   *We allow levels of water pollution that can cause gastrointestinal diseases, reproductive problems, neurological disorders, and cancer.*

◊   *We make lifestyle choices that have adverse health consequences. Excessive exposure to the sun can cause skin cancer. Lack of regular exercise can make us age faster and increase the risk and symptoms of more than twenty physical and mental-health conditions, including cancer, heart disease, dementia, stroke, type 2 diabetes, depression, obesity, and high blood pressure. Eating too much, especially of fatty, salty food, can lead to obesity, which is a risk factor for many diseases, among them diabetes, heart disease, osteoarthritis, sleep apnea, and even some cancers. Smoking harms heart and blood vessels in ways that make it a major risk factor for coronary heart disease, atherosclerosis, heart failure, and peripheral artery disease. Smoking is also a major risk factor for cancer, COPD, and diabetes. Chronic heavy drinking of alcohol can cause major health problems, including cirrhosis of the liver, anemia, cancer, cardiovascular disease, dementia, depression, seizures, gout, high blood pressure, infectious disease, nerve damage, and pancreatitis. Excessive drinking also encourages antisocial behaviors likely to lead to health-affecting accidents, such as car crashes, fights, falls, and the like. Risky behaviors make us more likely to get sexually transmitted diseases. Not washing our hands before meals puts us at risk for GI infections. Eating from buffets or open cafeteria lines makes us more likely to catch airborne diseases. Most pervasively, we make inadequate efforts to combat stress.*

◊   *A particularly negative health factor within our control is addiction, particularly opioid addiction. The 2016 Surgeon General's Report Facing Addiction in America estimates that 20.8 million Americans — 7.8% of the population — has a substance-use disorder. The report, first ever from the Surgeon General's office on addiction, conjectures that one of the reasons that this has become a problem is that substance abuse was traditionally treated as a social or criminal problem rather than a health problem, limiting prevention and treatment options.*

◊   *We accept public policy that discourages full participation in the health-care system by all Americans. The headline of the article of 6 April 2017 by Jessica Glenza in The Guardian says it all: "Rich Americans live up to 15 years longer than poor peers, studies find." Specifically, the article cites studies in The Lancet that examine how the American health system affects inequality, studies that conclude "the richest 1% live up to 15 years longer than the poorest 1%... a gap in life expectancy that has widened in recent decades, making poverty a powerful indicator for death." This is attributed to treating health care as a commodity rather than a right.*

What these failures mean and what should be done about them can be debated; but one conclusion that can be reliably drawn is there are things, both as individuals and as a society, we prize more than health for ourselves and our children.

Diseases That By Their Nature Are Difficult To Eradicate Or Cure

Even now, there remain types of diseases unlikely to be resolved in the foreseeable future through medical advances and technology. It's estimated that those least likely to be resolved include diseases of poverty, rare diseases, and cancer, as follows:

◊   *Diseases of Poverty*

Common Examples: Tuberculosis, malaria, HIV/AIDS, polio, measles, pertussis, diarrhoeal diseases, respiratory infections, malnutrition

According to Philip Stevens, Director of Health Projects, International Policy Network (IPN), "A large proportion of illnesses in low-income countries are entirely avoidable or treatable with existing medicines or interventions. Most of the disease burden in low-income countries finds its roots in the consequences of poverty, such as poor nutrition, indoor air pollution and lack of access to proper sanitation and health education. The WHO (World Health Organization) estimates that diseases associated with poverty account for 45 per cent of the disease burden in the poorest countries."

Why Rapid Resolution Is Unlikely: Poverty in low-income countries does not appear to be a currently pressing priority for other countries financially stable enough to address it. Also, political turmoil in some of the countries needing the most help hinders the effectiveness of outsiders who come to the country in an attempt to eradicate disease.

It should be pointed out that, even in the U.S., as economic disparities continue to drive increasing numbers of individuals and families into poverty, nutrition will suffer, which could lead to a growth in diseases in this category in the most-developed country in the world. Here, the failure to address the issue will probably stem from an ideological bias that assumes those suffering such diseases "deserve" them.

◊ ***Rare Diseases, sometimes called Orphan Diseases***

Description: A disease, often genetic in origin, that few people get.

Why Rapid Resolution Is Unlikely: So few people get the diseases that even a highly successful cure won't earn back the cost of R&D necessary to target the disease, which makes it difficult to get research backing. Occasionally, a cure for such a disease will be found as a byproduct of other research. Or an unexpected — and unique — publicity coup will get the disease more attention, as in 2014's challenge that went viral to raise over $115 million for ALS (amyotrophic lateral sclerosis, aka Lou Gehrig disease). The ALS Association promptly funneled the money into a global research initiative that has already identified a new gene, NEK1, that contributes to the disease.

◊   *Cancer: In the next few years, specific cancers may continue to be cured or controlled, but not cancer per se*

> ***Why Rapid Resolution Is Unlikely:*** Cancer is not one thing, but a class of illnesses characterized by unbounded cell replication that varies from cancer type to cancer type. What works to cure or control one cancer will not necessarily work for another.

The fact that much disease remains resistant to cure should not kill hope that a cure will be found. The interesting thing about disease resolution is that it can come almost out of the blue. As this is being written, an article in the *New York Times* is headlined "New Ebola Vaccine Gives 100 Percent Protection." Trials have been ongoing since 1976 with little result, but the 2014 epidemic that killed 11,000 people in Africa and spread overseas jumpstarted a new round of research, with the result that, just two years after the 2014 outbreak, there is a successful vaccine.

Antibiotic Resistance: Most Serious Setback In Modern Medicine

Penicillin, the first true antibiotic, was discovered by Scottish-born bacteriologist Alexander Fleming in 1928 and widely introduced in the 1940s. Because of his discovery, Fleming shared the 1945 Nobel Prize for Medicine with Australian pathologist Howard Walter Florey and German-born British biochemist Ernst Boris Chain, both of whom isolated and purified penicillin.

Since penicillin's discovery, over 100 antibiotics have come on the market, to be prescribed for an ever-widening range of bacteria-caused infections.

Antibiotics cure disease by attacking infection. While they do not work against virus-caused infections such as colds, the flu, bronchitis, viral gastroenteritis, and most coughs and sore throats, they are effective for infections caused by bacteria, fungi, and certain parasites.

Antibiotics are commonly prescribed following surgery and for open wounds. They are also prescribed for, among other conditions, sexually transmitted diseases, bacterial pneumonia, bacterial meningitis, staph, strep throat, and infections of the skin, urinary tract and eye. Antibiotics have literally been lifesavers, a long-taken-for-granted miracle banishing once-fatal or disfiguring diseases.

Their effectiveness led to antibiotics being over-used. It is common, for example, when alarming infection-type symptoms appear, for doctors to prescribe antibiotics as a safety measure even before tests confirm whether or not the infection is caused by bacteria or a virus. Adding to the problem is the fact that about 80% of all antibiotics used in the U.S. are administered in the agriculture industry, much of the use for nonmedical purposes such as promoting faster growth.

What this means is that, due to antibiotics being over-prescribed to people for three-quarters of a century and those same people eating food from animals subjected to massive antibiotics treatment, most Americans have been so over-exposed to antibiotics that almost everyone is at risk of being hit by an infection that has become antibiotic resistant.

Antibiotic-resistant bacteria have learned how, as the Centers for Disease Control and Prevention (CDC) puts it - "to outsmart the drugs." Bacteria do this by changing in a way that either (1) protects the bacteria from the drug or (2) neutralizes the drug. The resulting resistant bacteria multiply and spread, causing severe infections and sharing genetic information with other bacteria, making the other bacteria resistant as well. Each time this happens, treatment options become more limited and the number of untreatable infections grows. This is a particular problem for health-care facilities, where so-called "superbugs" are on the rise because even the most-powerful last-resort antibiotics are useless against them.

This is a huge step backward, and the resulting risk to public health is both major and real. The CDC estimates that two million Americans are infected with antibiotic-resistant bacteria each year and roughly 23,000 die. According to the Infectious Disease Society of America (IDSA), methicillin-resistant Staphylococcus aureus — aka MRSA — is alone responsible for more deaths annually than HIV/AIDS, Parkinson's, and homicide combined. The death toll will grow as bacteria now controlled by drugs grow resistant.

In "World faces decade at risk from antibiotic-resistant bugs," published in *The Guardian* December 30, 2016, health-focused philanthropist and tech titan Bill Gates pointed out that complacency following the success of antibiotics leaves the world at risk from untreatable pandemics capable of killing hundreds of thousands or even millions of people. At least some elected officials agree. Representative Tom Cole (R-OK), Chair, Subcommittee on Labor, HHS, Education and Related Agencies, said in the March 29, 2017, HHS budget hearing:

> *You're much more likely to die in a pandemic than you are in a terrorist attack... I'd much rather fight Ebola in West Africa than in West Dallas.*

A bioterrorist releasing antibiotic-resistant bacteria is probably the greatest potential security threat in the world today, especially since bacteria inhabit hosts that travel.

The remedies are few. Medicare uses the prevention approach, requiring hospitals and nursing homes to devise plans to (1) prevent the spread of drug-resistant infections and (2) limit the use of antibiotics to what is essential in specific situations. The CDC has adopted similar initiatives. The Food and Drug Administration (FDA) has simplified the process for antibiotic approval. The FDA also encourages the agricultural industry to limit the use of antibiotics in livestock. The

Biomedical Advanced Research and Development Authority (BARDA) focuses on the building of public-private partnerships for support of promising research. At least one executive order has been issued calling for across-the-board action against the threat.

According to Nicholas Bagley, law professor at the University of Michigan, and Kevin Outterson, law professor at Boston University and executive director of Carb-X (promoter of public-private partnerships against antibiotic resistance), the ultimately successful approach will be pharmaceutical in nature. Further, it may require a highly targeted strategy that will convince pharmaceutical companies to work on new antibiotics.

Developing new drugs is an expensive, time-consuming proposition, and what makes it worthwhile is the fact that, following approval of the drug, the FDA protects the developer of a new drug for a period of five to twelve years, which means that only the original developer or someone to whom that developer grants a license, can sell the drug during that period, further that no one else can sell a drug of an identical composition. Bagley and Outterson point out in an Op-Ed piece in *The New York Times* of January 18, 2017, that this approach works fine for most drugs that are approved, go to market, and are used in short order. For antibiotics, however, the usefulness of the approach is limited.

The reason is that new antibiotics are not used immediately, but are conserved as "drugs of last choice," employed only when older antibiotics have been tried and failed. This means that a new antibiotic may sit on the shelf for years. This limits the market so badly for so long that pharmaceutical companies do not see the development of antibiotics as a viable proposition. Instead, they work on drugs with more-immediate marketability. There have been laws that extend the "protected" period for antibiotics, but they do little to solve the problem.

Bagley and Outterson propose a novel solution: Congress "should reward manufacturers that bring a targeted, highly innovative antibiotic to market with a substantial financial prize (and) in exchange, manufacturers would surrender their patent."

This would remove the pressure on pharmaceutical companies to balance costs vs. likely profit when they decide to pursue development of a new antibiotic. Awarding such prizes would, Bagley and Outterson admit, be expensive:

> But you can't defeat bacteria on the cheap. They've survived for billions of years because they're so good at adapting to new threats. Staying one step ahead will require ingenuity, money and radical change. Tinkering around the margins isn't going to cut it.

They estimate the cost would be in the range of $4 billion a year, but it just might work, and it would be worth it.

The problem is being taken seriously. In September 2014, The White House issued *Executive Order - - Combating Antibiotic-Resistant Bacteria*. In this order,

President Obama called for "a strategic, coordinated, and sustained effort" to detect, prevent, and control antibiotic resistance.

The order identified this threat as a national-security priority and established the Task Force for Combating Antibiotic-Resistant Bacteria, to be co-chaired by the Secretaries of Defense, Agriculture, and Health and Human Services. The members include representatives from (1) the Departments of State, Justice, Veterans Affairs, and Homeland Security; (2) the Environmental Protection Agency; (3) the U.S. Agency for International Development; (4) the Office of Management and Budget; (5) the Domestic Policy Council; (6) the National Security Council staff; (7) the Office of Science and Technology Policy; and (8) the National Science Foundation. As recently as October 2016, the Centers for Disease Control and Prevention funded thirty-four new projects in support of this Task Force and other federal initiatives.

From this, it's clear that ambitious efforts are underway to tackle the problem. Let's hope that they succeed. Of all threats facing humans on earth, this is the one most likely to kill significant numbers of us literally overnight.

Chapter Ten.

Medical Error

When we go to a health-care provider, our highest hope is that we emerge cured. Our lowest expectation is that, cured or not, at least we will not be actively harmed while under the care of a doctor, nurse, or hospital. That expectation may be unfounded, and the "fly in the ointment" is medical error.

Frequency Of Medical Error

According to a landmark report published by the Institute of Medicine (IOM) in 1999, medical errors were then the third-leading cause of death in the U.S. The report, evidently the first of its kind, was considered shocking at the time. Subsequent studies, however, have suggested that this number may be on the low side, although many in the medical profession dispute the methodologies used in defining "medical error."

What's Included In "Medical Error"

There is little disagreement that, as Martin Makary and Michael Daniel of Johns Hopkins University School of Medicine contend in their *BMJ (British Medical Journal)* article of 2013, "error" should include:

◊ *An unintended act (either of commission or omission)*

◊ *The failure of a planned action to be completed (an error of execution)*

◊ *The use of a wrong plan to achieve an aim (an error of planning)*

◊ *Deviation from the process of care (either of commission or omission)*

It seems too broad, however, to include "an act that does not achieve its intended outcome." Does that element not incorporate other factors — such as the cumulative impact of patient lifestyle choices — over which health-care providers have no control and oftentimes inadequate knowledge when they decide on a course of treatment?

A particularly worrisome form of medical error is that defined by the National Quality Forum (NQF) as a "Never Event" — that is, an error in medical care that is clearly identifiable, preventable, and serious in its consequences for the patient. According to the NQF, "never events" indicate basic problems in a facility's safety and credibility.

Why Medical Error Doesn't Show Up As A Cause Of Death

Even though it's estimated that preventable medical errors claim the lives of probably between 210,000 and 400,000 Americans each year, which would put error third behind only heart disease and cancer as a cause of death, medical errors don't appear on the CDC's "Leading Causes of Death" list.

In their 2013 *BMJ* article, Makary and Daniel contend that the reason that medical error doesn't show up as a leading cause of death is because there's no easy way to code human and system factors as a cause. They say there's no place, for example, to put medical error as a cause on U.S. death certificates, and also that ICD (International Classification of Disease) codes do not include medical error as a death cause. This means that typically the cause of death will be assigned to the underlying condition that brought the patient into the health-care system even if that condition is not the immediate reason the patient died.

Most-Common Medical Errors

There are various kinds of medical errors. Some of the more obvious that come to mind are:

◊   *Failure to order appropriate medical tests or imaging studies*

◊   *Misreading medical tests or imaging studies*

◊   *Failing to incorporate the results of medical tests or imaging studies when diagnosing or making treatment plans*

◊   *Performing surgery on the wrong part of the body*

◊   *Making a mistake in surgical technique*

◊   *Leaving foreign objects in the body during surgery*

◊   *Prescribing or administering incorrect medication*

◊   *Failing to follow treatment plans*

◊   *Failing to maintain proper hygiene*

◊   *Miscommunicating with the growing number of American patients who do not speak English as their primary language*

— according to U.S. census data released in 2015, over 25 million Americans self-identify as having limited English proficiency (This is a provider issue because Title VI of the Civil Rights Act of 1964 has been ruled to incorporate protections against discrimination based on national origin and language.)

The Dunning-Kruger Effect — Operating At The Edge of Competence

Take error a step further to the Dunning-Kruger effect — what might be termed deception or even self-deception — in which an institution or its personnel or vendors operate at the edge of competence or beyond and understand so little about certain conditions or situations that they don't know what they don't know. When this failure to assess expertise properly is incorporated into hospital marketing, the consequences can be significant. As this was being written, for example, a jury in Jefferson County, Alabama, awarded $16 million to a Mountain Brook couple suing a local medical center because of damages suffered during delivery of the couple's fourth child. Five million dollars of the award represented punitive damages for reckless fraud related to an advertising and marketing campaign that misrepresented the hospital's expertise in and approach to natural childbirth. While the amount of the award will probably be appealed, the essential outcome is likely to be upheld because, according to the plaintiffs' counsel, the marketing campaign wasn't reviewed by the hospital's medical staff or subjected to its internal fraud-review process.

Provider Failure To Admit Error

Compounding the problem of medical error is that providers often do not admit that something went wrong. Even after it becomes clear that there is a new problem, the provider may refuse to divulge information relating to the issue. This means that information that might help patients get appropriate treatment for ongoing problems related to the error may be withheld.

When a mistake is made, the victims and their survivors can expect little help from authorities. It is states that have the power to legislate issues relating to medical liability, and, according to ProPublica.org in "A Trail of Medical Errors Ends in Grief, But No Answers" by Marshall Allen and Olga Pierce (Dec. 18, 2015):

> *Only 10 states require hospitals to disclose medical mistakes or unintended outcomes to patients. More than two-thirds of states have laws granting legal immunity for apologies by providers. But apologies aren't required, and the laws on immunity often do not shield doctors from liability if they explain what went wrong.*

What it comes down to is that providers feel there is so much legal advantage in keeping quiet about error that they are reluctant to admit what has happened

— even when, ethically, they would be more comfortable doing so. Ironically, the experience of the few hospitals that have "coming clean" policies suggests that, in the long run, they may have less difficulty if they quickly admit error and make sensible restitution to victims and/or their survivors.

The prevailing hospital policy of concealing error forces victims and/or their survivors who want to learn what happened to sue, complain to state regulatory agencies, or turn to professional associations or monitoring organizations like The Joint Commission, the nonprofit organization that accredits most hospitals. None of these actions is guaranteed to produce any more information. Unless there's a "smoking gun" — a paper trail or an inside whistleblower — it's unlikely that a lawsuit will prevail. Regulators often refuse to investigate unless they feel an issue of broader patient safety is involved; and, even when they do investigate, may keep the details confidential. The Joint Commission has an online form for reporting "a new patient safety event or concern" but states on its "Report a Patient Safety Event" page only that:

◊   *We check for other patient safety events about the organization.*

◊   *We may write to the organization about your concern.*

◊   *Sometimes, we visit the organization to see if there is a problem in meeting the requirements that deal with your concern.*

In essence, according to current law and custom, those harmed by medical error have little recourse to remedy and may never learn exactly what happened.

AHRQ Quality Indicators

Rather than ignoring or attempting to explain away error, the best hospitals undertake to avoid it. Understanding the precise nature of error is the beginning of addressing the issue. Government policy is to offer support to hospitals trying to improve, and to that end the Agency for Healthcare Research and Quality (AHRQ) has published quality and safety indicators to enable consistent identification of error.

To aid hospitals planning to use its Quality Indicators "to track and improve inpatient quality and patient safety," AHRQ issues a toolkit that includes modules measuring hospital quality and safety relative to (1) patient safety indicators (PSIs); (2) inpatient quality indicators (IQIs); and (3) pediatric quality indicators (PDIs), as well as general usage information and free software hospitals can use to apply the indicators to their discharge data. Hospital interest in using PSIs is intensifying because they are key indicators for CMS programs comparing institutional quality.

Who Pays For Medical Error?

Adding insult to injury, unless there is clear proof, which usually means a paper trail or an insider willing to testify on the patient's behalf, it is generally the patient or the patient's insurance plan that pays for any treatment caused by error. This is a significant amount of money annually. According to an article of January 16, 2016, in HealthNetwork, "in 2008, which is the last year the problem was studied in terms of cost, medical errors added an extra cost of $19.5 billion dollars in national spending."

On the bright side, some hospitals have now instituted a policy requiring that patients be told when a medical error has occurred and what caused it, if known. In those hospitals – unfortunately still just a relative handful – the hospital will usually cover costs for any follow-up care needed due to the error. The "honesty is the best policy" approach is, again according to the HealthNetwork, supported by the AMA, the federal Agency for Healthcare Research and Quality, the American College of Obstetricians and Gynecologists, and The Leapfrog Organization, which has become the foremost organization grading hospitals for various quality components, including error.

Impact Of Medical Error

While there may be disagreement as to the frequency of error— and some within the medical community claim that error is underreported – mistakes drive up the cost of health care for payers and cause harm to patients, probably why both payers and patients are demanding more transparency from hospitals as to quality and safety.

Chapter Eleven.

Outcomes for Patients, Providers, Payers

In the current health-care environment, there are both positive and negative outcomes for patients, providers, and payers.

On The Positive Side
On the positive side from the perspective of these three constituencies:

◊　*Patients in the U.S. have access to an increasing range of generally more-effective health procedures and products.*

◊　*Providers enjoy large built-in demand and can access an increasing range of products and procedures to satisfy it. Nurses, physicians, and pharmacists are at the top of the list of occupations most trusted by the American public.*

◊　*Payers operate in a decreasingly competitive environment, have the clout to negotiate provider rates vigorously, and face relatively ineffective resistance to premium-rate increases. Evolving algorithms should make it easier to spot health-care fraud.*

On The Negative Side:
On the negative side from the perspective of these three constituencies:

◊　*Patients as a group find themselves paying more out-of-pocket costs in the form of higher co-pays and deductibles even as they feel less of a personal connection to their caregivers. Patients are sometimes denied ongoing access not only to new drugs but also to drugs they've used for years because they can't afford the increased prices that follow sale of the drug to a pharmaceutical or other company with a "whatever the market will bear" business model. Patients continue to be subject to an unacceptable amount of medical error.*

◊　*Providers are under intense pressure from payers to offer increasingly higher quality care in a more cost-effective environment beset by change. This leads to physicians spending more time on administration and compliance and less with patients. This is a source of great frustration for many in the profession, in part because it undermines their personal satisfaction in the healing process. Less time with patients also interferes with patient relations because physicians in that position exert less authority with patients who require intensive attention from their doctors in order to respect their judgment. The latter condition is known as HLOC (Health Locus of Control) and is increasingly recognized as being critical in having patients follow doctors' orders. Hospitals find their traditional role undermined as payers promote the use of smaller, less expensive, specialized-function facilities. As for nurses, the most numerous health-care profession as well as the most respected among members of the general public, many feel micromanaged, unappreciated, and too often used as guinea pigs for change by their employers.*

◊   *Payers in the private-insurance sector have had their business models upended by provisions in the 2010 ACA that in essence remove some of the strategies they've always used to keep profits high. This is happening even as "what the market will bear" drug pricing is prompting them to reassess their formularies in ways that make their customers distrust them. They are also beset by more-sophisticated forms of medical fraud.*

How Does The U.S. Stack Up?

In spite of the fact that the U.S. spends so much on health care, outcomes are among the worst in the developed world. As a general population, we die sooner and are more likely to suffer from chronic conditions than do our cohorts in other high-income countries. In 2012, life at expectancy at birth in these countries was as follows:

◊   *83.10 years*   *Japan*

◊   *81.50 years*   *U.K.*

◊   *78.74 years*   *USA*

This is partly because of unhealthy lifestyle choices: overeating; lack of exercise; continuing tobacco use; excessive alcohol use; drug abuse; and the like. There is also, however, a failure to apply public-health concepts to chronic-disease management, as well as a lack of coordination in health care that makes error and oversight more likely than in nations with more coordinated health-care delivery models. The most disturbing aspect of the life-expectancy comparison between the U.S. and other countries is that we are falling further behind and are expected to head even lower. A study from *The Lancet,* one of the most respected medical journals in the world, which was reported in *The Guardian* (21 February 2017), anticipates that "life expectancy will soon exceed 90 years for the first time." Here's the study's list of developed nations, with approximate life-expectancy-at-birth estimates for female babies born in 2030:

◊ *#1 - South Korea - 90.8 years (men can look forward to 84.1)*

◊ *#2 - France - 88 years*

◊ *#3 - Japan - 88 years*

◊ *#4 - Switzerland - 87 years*

◊ *#5 - Australia - 87 years*

◊ *#6 - Ireland - 86 years*

◊ *#7 - Germany - 86 years*

◊ *#8 - U.K. - 86 years*

◊ *#9 - U.S. - 83.3 years for women (men can look forward to 79.5)*

South Korea has made big health strides due to economic improvement, educational attainment, decrease in death from infectious diseases, and improved nutrition. Also, obesity — a risk factor for several serious chronic diseases — has not become a major problem, and the number of women who smoke remains relatively low. Why does the U.S. fare so poorly when compared to other industrialized nations? The study notes that the U.S. is "the only country in the Organisation for Economic Cooperation and Development without universal healthcare coverage."

There are significant differences among American states as to life expectancies at birth. According to The Henry J. Kaiser Family Foundation (basing its statistics on CDC numbers), here's a sampling from 2009, showing the top and bottom of the list in terms of how long a baby is likely to live in each state:

◊ *81.3 years*   *Hawaii*

◊ *81.1 years*   *Minnesota*

◊ *80.8 years*   *California, Connecticut*

◊ *80.5 years*   *Massachusetts, New York, Vermont*

◊ *80.3 years*   *New Hampshire, New Jersey*

◊   80.2 years   *Utah*

◊   80.0 years   *Colorado, Wisconsin*

◊   75.9 years   *Oklahoma*

◊   75.7 years   *Louisiana*

◊   75.4 years   *Alabama, West Virginia*

◊   75.0 years   *Mississippi*

Those babies born in the states at the head of the list are anticipated at the time of their birth to live to be over the age of eighty, those born in the states at the bottom to be less than seventy-six when they die. That's a significant difference that probably relates to diet, climate, drug use, smoking, exercise, other lifestyle factors, and availability of affordable health services.

Nationwide, life expectancy goes up as people age and the age-at-death difference between women and men diminishes. For example, in 2013, the Social Security Administration published an actuarial table showing these life expectancies for Americans:

◊   *At age 25, American males can expect to live another 52.47 years and American females another 56.85, making males 77.47 and females 81.85 at estimated time of death, a difference between the sexes of 4.38 years.*

◊   *At age 50, American males can expect to live another 29.58 years and American females another 33.16, making males 79.58 and females 83.16 at estimated time of death, a difference between the sexes of 3.58 years.*

◊   *At age 75, American males can expect to live another 11.03 years and American females another 12.83, making males 86.03 and females 87.83 at estimated time of death, a difference between the sexes of 1.8 years.*

◊   *At age 90, American males can expect to live another 4.03 years and American females another 4.80, making males 94.03 and females 94.80 at estimated time of death, a difference between the sexes of .77 years.*

Many variables affect life expectancy. Given what the U.S. spends on health care, however, it is surprising how poor our life expectancy is when compared to that of the citizens of other industrialized nations around the globe.

Outcomes As A Driver Of What's Happening In The Provider Universe

American health care as traditionally practiced has led to unsustainable costs, especially given the number of Baby Boomers either already in or about to enter Medicare and thus at the time of their lives when, typically, their need for medical services increases. Other factors in exploding costs have to do with:

◊ *Medical error*

◊ *The use of expensive advanced technologies*

◊ *The development of treatments for once-fatal chronic diseases*

◊ *The ability to extend life indefinitely*

◊ *The failure of patients who don't want certain kinds of medical care to execute living wills*

◊ *The demand for higher profits from shareholders in pharmaceutical and insurance companies*

What made the growth in health-care costs particularly unacceptable was that quality not only did not keep up with costs, but also compared poorly with that of other developed nations that spend less on health care.

It is this payer and patient dissatisfaction with American health-care outcomes and costs that is propelling the changes currently roiling The Provider Universe, changes so profound that they amount to a revolution.

PART TWO.
THE PROVIDER UNIVERSE

Chapter Twelve.

Why It Sometimes Seems As If The American Health-Care System Is Set Up To Benefit Everyone But Patients

Most of the time, today's health-care system works to benefit the patient to a degree unthinkable just a few years ago, yet many patients — and not just those whose outcomes are less than outstanding — are puzzled, frustrated, dissatisfied, or even angry with their experience.

This isn't surprising. When an individual enters today's system, it is often in circumstances bordering on panic. The familiar world in which health is taken for granted rapidly dissolves into a there-be-dragons universe in which a patient seems to become no more than a collection of symptoms to be measured, categorized, and made money off of.

At best, this landscape can be confusing to navigate. At worst, it can be so personally dismissive as to seem populated with combatants who, for purposes of their own, use rules and processes to overwhelm and exploit all who enter.

The principal reasons for this disconnect between actual patient benefit and perceived disregard for patients relate to (1) the size of the health-care industry, (2) patient attitudes toward health care and their role in it, (3) publicity given unusual patient experiences, good and bad , and (4) the revolution the industry is undergoing.

A quick look at these factors will show how each influences perceptions of health care.

Health Care Is Big Business

The individual patient is a speck in a large medical landscape. According to the Bureau of Labor Statistics (BLS), in 2014 the "Health care and social assistance" subset of the "Services-providing sector" employed 18,057,400 and by 2024 is expected to employ 21,852,200. This made the health-care industry the third largest employer in the U.S. in 2014, just behind "State and local government" and "Professional and business services." The 2024 projection, if met, will make health care the largest employer in the U.S.

This is *big* business. In 2014 approximately $3.0 trillion was spent on health care in the United States, 17.5% of the Gross National Product. By 2024, it's estimated that the amount of such spending will increase to 19.6%, which means that almost $1 of every $5 spent in the U.S. will be for health care. Among developed countries internationally, the U.S. is the big spender. With that much money at stake, you can safely bet that some bizarre things happen on the way to the bank.

The net result is a system broken into many pieces that have not traditionally viewed themselves as collectively responsible for patient care. Rather, they operate as individual entities balancing their financial needs with their responsibilities to *one aspect* of patient care. This can give the impression that each time a patient sees a new provider, even if the visit is part of an ongoing health situation, he or she is "starting over." Even when seeing a long-time provider for a new condition, there's often a sense that the patient has no history of prior health care.

When patients seek assistance from any part of this system, they become customers as well as recipients of care. When compared to other industries, health-care customer-service protocols look, and often are, more compassionate and individualized, even within the largest providers. At the same time, as in any big business, the needs and wishes of individual customers are but one of many competing priorities.

It is the "squeaking wheel that gets the grease," and there are many factors out there capable of squeaking much louder in The Provider Universe than the individual in the throes of a personal health crisis. This can make it seem as if patients don't matter.

The Role Of The Patient In Shaping Health Care

As the basic component, patients are a primary driver of the health-care system in that (1) our expectations provide an excuse for much of what's done and (2) our habits and choices make much of it necessary.

Patient Expectations Of Health Care

Our expectation is that, if we or our insurance plan is willing to pay for it, everything possible will be done to correct or significantly ameliorate the condition or disease that brought us into the system. And publicity surrounding diagnostic advances, miracle drugs, and innovative surgeries leads us to think that just about anything is possible in terms of both treatment and outcome.

Ever optimistic, we are unwilling to accept health-related limitations if medicine can make us better, and most of us, at least at the outset of a condition, believe that medicine can. Forty years ago, for example, patients with cataracts accepted that, following surgery, their eyesight would be somewhat improved. Today, that'd be a fail.

How fast the medical miracle will be worked on our behalf matters. Both we and our friends, families, and employers expect that we will get back to normal quickly and without complications.

If we don't get the result we expect within what we consider a reasonable time frame, we are more likely to make waves, file complaints, leave bad online reviews, or even sue. Negativity builds on negativity, and patient perceptions of their importance in the health-care system continue to deteriorate.

Patient Habits & Lifestyle Choices

Our health-affecting habits are more likely to "get us" now than in our grand-parents' day. We travel internationally more often, potentially not only acquiring but bringing home once-exotic diseases and new viruses. We are heavier, get less physical exercise, eat fattier diets, and are subject to greater societal stress. We are likely to be more socially isolated than we would have been a generation ago.

Certain of our lifestyle choices are more dangerous than others, particularly smoking and excessive drinking.

As recently as 2014, the last year for which numbers are available, the Centers for Disease Control and Prevention (CDC) estimates that 40 million adults in the U.S. smoke cigarettes and more than 16 million Americans live with a smoking-related disease. While many diseases may or may not be smoking-related, some of those that can definitely be caused and/or worsened by smoking include:

◊ *Cancer of the bladder, esophagus, larynx, lung, mouth, throat, cervix, kidney, pancreas, and stomach*

◊ *Chronic lung disease*

◊ *Chronic heart and cardiovascular disease*

◊ *Chronic bronchitis and chronic obstructive pulmonary disease (COPD)*

◊ *Acute myeloid leukemia*

◊ *Abdominal aortic aneurysm*

◊ *Cataracts*

◊ *Periodontitis*

◊ *Pneumonia*

◊ *Reproductive problems*

In 2004, U.S. Surgeon General Richard Carmona said that smokers die thirteen to fourteen years before nonsmokers.

The CDC offers a similarly depressing picture for excessive alcohol use, citing short-term health risks of injuries, violence, alcohol poisoning, risky sexual behaviors, and miscarriage and stillbirth. As for long-term alcohol-related health risks, they include the development of both fatal and chronic diseases, learning and memory problems, mental-health problems, social problems, and alcoholism. The CDC estimates that excessive alcohol use can shorten life span by as much as thirty years and in recent years has been responsible for as many as one in ten deaths in the U.S., while cigarette smoking accounts for one of every five deaths. This means that roughly three of every ten deaths in the U.S. is a more-or-less direct result of just these two habits.

While bad eating habits may not be as obvious a health risk, in the long run they have the power to be even more lethal because more widespread. Nutritional deficiencies can cause or exacerbate illness. As for obesity, it increases the risk for coronary heart disease, high blood pressure, stroke, type 2 diabetes, cancer, osteoarthritis, sleep apnea, obesity hypoventilation syndrome, reproductive problems, and gallstones.

In connection with the issue of patient habits, the choice of where and how we live, our driving habits, and the jobs we hold should be mentioned.

Much of what we're talking about here relates to environmental issues, particularly air and water pollution. Health effects related to air pollution include:

◊ *Respiratory diseases, such as asthma and changes in lung function*

◊ *Cardiovascular diseases*

◊ *Adverse pregnancy outcomes*

◊ *Death*

In 2013 the International Agency for Research on Cancer (IARC) of the World Health Organization (WHO) concluded that "outdoor air pollution is carcinogenic to humans, with the particulate matter component of air pollution most closely associated with increased cancer incidence, especially cancer of the lung." The IARC also noted an association between outdoor air pollution and increase in cancer of the urinary tract/bladder. Indoor air pollution, usually related to poor ventilation and use of noxious cleaning supplies, can cause many of the same health issues.

Health effects related to water pollution include:

◊ *Infectious diseases, such as typhoid, cholera, paratyphoid fever, dysentery, jaundice, amoebiasis, and malaria — caused by water contaminated by sewage, chemical spills, and the like*

◊ *Damage to the nervous system and cancer — caused by the carbonates and organophosphates that pesticides contain*

◊ *Reproductive and endocrinal damage – caused by chlorides*

◊ *Restriction to the amount of oxygen in the brain – caused by nitrates*

◊ *Damage to the central nervous system – caused by lead accumulation*

◊ *Liver damage, skin cancer and vascular diseases – caused by arsenic*

◊ *Damage to the spinal cord – caused by excessive fluorides*

◊ *Cancer – caused by petrochemicals*

It's impossible to avoid all contact with air and water pollution, but some geographic areas and occupations are more affected than others. Individuals living in those areas and/or working in those occupations are more likely to get the diseases associated with pollution.

Patient Disconnect

Because of its seemingly arbitrary and somewhat opaque nature, many of us have fallen into the habit of assuming the health-care system will work its magic independently of our involvement (apart from providing our bodies for it to practice on). We usually prefer the silver bullet of fast and drastic health-provider action to making long-term changes in our health-affecting habits, especially if they're part of a lifestyle that we enjoy.

This lack of "ownership in the process" probably arises from several factors. For one thing, patients have traditionally not been held accountable for taking action to improve their health. If patient failure to follow doctor's orders resulted in the need for ongoing treatment, not only did doctors continue to provide the care but insurance companies paid for it. Probably the second most important factor in not assuming ownership for the process is the fact that those of us with insurance, including Medicare and Medicaid, never pay directly for the full amount billed for services and products, but only for any co-pays or deductibles.

Adding to patient disconnect is the potential conflict between perception and reality. What we are convinced that we need may not improve our condition. At the same time, health-care providers have an ethical responsibility to address needs more than preferences, which may lead them to subject us to therapies whose value we don't recognize.

A related perception issue is the need for the health-care system to convince us as patients that we are receiving *appropriate* care. We must feel not only that our health is improved, but that we received the latest and greatest from expert professionals in an up-to-the-minute environment. Further, we tend to expect this whether or not access to that level of facility and service affects outcomes in a specific situation. This means that even a successful outcome will not necessarily satisfy patients that they received what they think they were entitled to in any given health event.

Finally, let's admit that there is something ultimately reassuring about trusting the health-care system enough so that we see ourselves going into it wounded by accident or enfeebled by illness and coming out mended or cured without ever having to consider what made that possible. In this scenario, our feeling seems to be that "as long as it works, I shouldn't have to think about it."

That attitude may serve well enough in eras of stability and lack of change, but it can leave patients at a disadvantage in more turbulent times, like today.

Publicity Given Health Care, Good & Bad

Social media and its relentless demand for continually refreshed data have turned most of us into newshounds, and all outlets search nonstop for interesting stories to feed a seemingly insatiable need. Patients whose lives have been changed forever by health care are among the most interesting. Sometimes the changes have been miraculous, sometimes catastrophic. Either way, we read about them with bated breath, experiencing at second hand what they experienced. The catastrophic experiences make us suspicious of health care, wondering if the next newsworthy medical error will be one committed on our persons, even though such errors are unlikely to happen to us. The miraculous experiences make us assume that, with modern medicine, all things are possible — whatever we manage to do to ourselves, health care can handle it. This impression of "medicine can do anything" is reinforced by all the publicity given medical advances and new health-care technologies. Neither suspicion nor complacency, while understandable, is statistically realistic when it comes to health care.

The Revolution The Industry Is Undergoing

The Provider Universe is undergoing its most massive transformation ever. Driven by medical advances, payer resistance to costs, legislation, regulation, competition, and changing patient expectations and attitudes, this transformation is affecting or will soon affect:

◊ *Where, how, and when health care is delivered*

◊ *How health-care providers will be rewarded (or penalized) for the patient outcomes they deliver*

◊ *How health-care services and products will be billed and paid*

◊ *Who will have the upper hand in continuum-of-care arrangements involving several providers attending to a patient's health*

◊   *Whether payers will continue to pay for all provider services or just those with proven positive impact*

◊   *How much responsibility patients will be expected to assume for the management of their health*

Patients and their health are the rationale for this massive industry, but so many other issues are in turmoil that we may sometimes seem like an afterthought.

Major Challenges & Major Players

While there's a lot going on in different parts of The Provider Universe, there are major developments and issues that challenge the overall status quo and significantly affect patient care. These are:

◊   *Medical advances and new technology*

◊   *Information technology*

◊   *Emerging care-delivery models and reimbursement*

◊   *Patient empowerment*

◊   *The political-football factor*

These and other issues have specific effects on those parts of The Provider Universe that play the greatest role in shaping patient care:

◊   *Physicians*

◊   *Hospitals*

◊   *Nurses*

To get a better grip on what patients need to do to remain the center of attention, whatever is going on, it's helpful to have at least a general understanding of these major challenges and players.

Chapter Thirteen.

Major Challenge: Medical Advances & New Technology

Now that we've done a quick flyover of the American health-care landscape (**Part One.** *American Health Care*), let's look at certain parts of it piece by piece. We'll start with what's coming in medical advances and new technology and the challenges this poses for The Provider Universe.

Significant as are the advances in medicine in the last few decades (See **Chapter Eight.** *Medical Advances, Medical Miracles*), some truly breathtaking developments lie ahead: some already in their infancy; some on the horizon; and some envisioned as a logical outcome of current knowledge and techniques.

Summary Of Noteworthy Medical Advances & New Technology

Every part of medicine will be affected by medical advances and new technologies. Some developments target diagnostics, providing either more-accurate diagnostics or diagnostics that were not previously possible. Other developments make it possible to correct conditions once fatal or leading to disability. Some stop or — it's anticipated at some point — reverse the aging process. Other developments will make health-care fraud more difficult.

Here are some of the buzzwords you'll hear in the years ahead and what they mean for health care.

◊ *Advanced MRI scanning can "see" diseases that cannot be accurately confirmed in any other way.*

◊ *A revolutionary blood test known as a liquid biopsy — already used in non-invasive prenatal tests for Down's syndrome — will detect the recurrence of cancer up to a year before it is detectable by other means, giving doctors critical extra time to fight the recurrence. The test also evaluates the effectiveness of chemotherapy. The test does this by detecting free-floating mutated DNA released into the bloodstream by dying cancer cells.*

◊　　*Artificial intelligence (AI) is the use of computer technology to analyze symptoms and compile treatment plans faster and with greater accuracy. The use of artificial intelligence to support physician decision-making will be taught as a primary topic in medical schools.*

◊　　*Augmented reality is a real-world environment enhanced by computer-generated sensory input (sound, video, graphics, etc.). In medicine, it is used for patient-care management via wearable devices, simulation in medical-training settings, and conducting complex surgeries. A particularly useful application relates to clinical trials that will use tiny microchips as models of human cells, organs, or whole physiological systems to substitute individualized computer simulation for the testing of medical products or interventions, thus doing away with the need for long and expensive trials that require human and/or animal testing.*

◊　　*Behavior monitors in the form of tiny, digestible sensors will be able to transmit condition-related data to caregivers.*

◊　　*Biometric identifiers are physiological characteristics unique to the individual – DNA, fingerprints, palm prints, iris patterns, and the like. They will be used to authenticate access to treatment.*

◊　　*Electronic health records (EHRs) are the digital repository for all information relating to an individual's health care throughout life. They are meant to be available to the patient and all members of his or her caregiver chain 24/7. When their compilation is matured as contemplated, they will include not only medical information specific to the individual (exam and testing results, treatment plans, outcomes, etc.) but also information provided by the patient as to personal life-style and other factors affecting health, as well as information relating the individual to a population-health cohort.*

◊　　*Medical 3D printing uses bioink based on the individual's own body chemistry to create organs and other body parts needed for transplantation or other aspects of patient care.*

◊　　*Medical robotics is the broad term given technologies that can create machines and devices (1) capable of performing tasks related to patient care or (2) substituting for damaged body parts. In the first category, for example, are robots that could be used to move patients, deliver supplies, etc. Also in the first category are nanorobots too small to be seen by the naked eye that can be introduced into a patient's bloodstream to perform highly targeted surgeries or drug therapies. In the second category are devices like the newly announced silicon-based robotic sleeve that mimics heart muscle to help hearts pump when they are failing.*

◊ *Multi-function radiology will be able to detect, simultaneously, a variety of medical problems, biomarkers, and symptoms without the need for additional tests.*

◊ *Optogenetics — the use of light to control cells in living tissue and thus to influence functions such as memory — is capable of supporting barely glimpsed advances, perhaps the most intriguing of which is the generation of false memories of taking drugs such as painkillers, tranquilizers, and stimulants. Given the placebo effect, this could radically alter reliance on the drugs most often abused.*

◊ *Precision medicine — derived from individual variability in genes, environment, and lifestyle — will offer an increasingly personalized approach to diagnosis and treatment. This use of genetics/genomics will revolutionize patient care.*

◊ *Virtual reality (VR) is the term used for computer-generated images that either replicate a real environment or create an imaginary one into which the user can enter. In health care, VR is used for medical training and education — virtual dissection tables and surgery simulators, for example. In clinical settings, VR is used for exposure therapy, pain management. brain-damage assessment and rehabilitation, social cognition training for young adults with autism, and the like.*

Perhaps the advances that will have the most overall impact will be those relating to communications, research, recordkeeping, and care delivery that will combine to empower patients so that they can and will assume a significantly more-active role in the management of their health care.

Not all changes in health care are, however, positive. Sometimes, as pointed out in **Chapter Nine.** *Medical And System Failures*, health care actually moves backwards. Antibiotic resistance, to take the primary example, is the most serious setback in modern medicine. Caused by overuse and misuse of antibiotics in people and the animals whose products they consume, antibiotic resistance has the potential to create a situation in which an untreatable bacteria kills hundreds of thousands or even millions of people in short order. Even now, in the absence of a wide-scale epidemic, it's estimated that over 23,000 people die annually in the U.S. due to antibiotic resistance. The only answers are (1) prevention— particularly attention to hygiene, especially in health-care settings — and (2) new antibiotics to which bacteria have not yet developed immunity. In spite of the fact that this is probably the most-critical issue facing medicine today, there seems to be relatively little pharmaceutical research underway because the profit potential is low.

Significance For The Provider Universe

On the positive side, providers - especially doctors and hospitals - have an additional weapon in their arsenals of care with which to help patients. New fields of specialization made possible by advances will open up to doctors, APRNs, and other professionals, increasing the number of jobs. Also, providers have another product or service to sell to help their bottom line.

On the negative side, not all advances live up to their potential. Also, each advance requires training and/or retraining, investment in upgraded facilities, and the risk of employing something new in its early stages before the provider has a handle on those most likely to benefit from or be harmed by its use. Advances will not benefit all patients equally, if at all, and not all patients will welcome or even willingly accept what will be required to access diagnostics and treatments based on genetics/genomics.

Payers will benefit when advances limit or end the need for ongoing care. They will, however, find themselves confronted by providers offering an almost limitless array of treatment options and patients wanting hugely expensive treatments that may or may not benefit them. This will be a particular issue for the chronically ill.

Patients will benefit from increasingly sophisticated capabilities that will enhance both fitness and longevity to an unparalleled degree. At the same time, they must be prepared to sacrifice a certain amount of personal privacy in order to access the most-advanced care that can mean the difference between life vs. death and function vs. disability.

Probably the greatest significance of advances will be the growth of an ethical debate that will become more contentious over time. Whether patients, providers, or payers, both as individuals and as members of a larger society, we will be forced to ask ourselves uncomfortable questions. Should medical treatment be equal for all or should it be allocated according to various factors such as efficacy, patient age and willingness to accept personal responsibility for health, and/or cost and patient ability to pay? Should every treatment possibility be applied in every situation or only in those where it's more likely to work? When do the positive effects of individual health improvement and life prolongation begin to be outweighed by the associated costs? The ultimate question, of course, is what is the true purpose of medicine? How much medicine is enough?

The Bottom Line

Every medical advance and each piece of new technology carries with it both positives and negatives for The Provider Universe, the payers that support it, and the patients who enter it.

We are entering a world in which what was before only a product of science fiction is becoming reality in that we will be able to use precision medicine to keep ourselves alive indefinitely. The "us" we are keeping alive isn't the original model, of course, but a patched-together version that is a facsimile. That seems worth doing as long as our minds are viable, for it is what is in our heads that makes us unique beings. That makes it even more imperative that medical advances include something capable of either (1) curing Alzheimers and other mental ailments or (2) giving us a timeline for when our minds will go. Of course, if we haven't written living wills, providers will likely keep us alive as long as our insurance holds out, even if we are merely enduring.

In the end, it comes down to the big payers — government programs and insurance companies — for only they will have the resource that will be required for this "life with almost no limit."

Even miracles have tradeoffs.

Chapter Fourteen.

Major Challenge: Information Technology

Merriam-Webster defines information technology (IT) as "the technology involving the development, maintenance, and use of computer systems, software, and networks for the processing and distribution of data." Health information technology (HIT) refers to IT employed within and/or for the purposes of health care.

Payers — insurance companies, employers with their own health plans, and government programs like Medicare and Medicaid — generally adopted HIT as quickly as possible because it simplified the handling of claims and also because they could afford the expensive new systems. Some providers, especially large hospitals and medical practices, were eager, early adopters of whatever benefit that HIT could bring to their processes and procedures. Others implemented it piecemeal. Procrastination was permissible because the rate of adoption was voluntary.

Overall, The Provider Universe was slow to adopt HIT, and it was perceived that this procrastination was a primary reason for poor outcomes and accelerating costs. The lack of ongoing, accurate digital records meant that a patient's medical history was buried piecemeal in either paper files or an assortment of often incompatible software programs in various provider offices, inaccessible and sometimes even unsuspected by the patient's other providers. This could lead to diagnosis based on incomplete information, treatment that might duplicate or even counter earlier treatment, and lack of vital information as to allergies or drug reactions.

For patients, this meant that records could be accessed only with difficulty and also that records could vary greatly from provider to provider in the degree and nature of detail provided.

From payer perspectives, this piecemeal recordkeeping encouraged billing for duplicated services. There was even a public-health issue in that piecemeal recordkeeping made it easier for patients to access drugs in inappropriate quantities, leading to abuse or illegal sale. In fact, for all involved in the health-care spectrum — patients, providers, and payers — piecemeal recordkeeping meant inefficiencies and a greater possibility of error.

Summary Of Issues Relating To Information Technology

Procrastination as to HIT ceased being optional following several pieces of legislation making rules and setting deadlines for its "meaningful use" across The Provider Universe. Below is a list of pertinent federal legislation, together with a brief description of those parts of the legislation affecting HIT and dates.

◊   *Health Insurance Portability and Accountability Act of 1996 (HIPAA) gave patients rights over their health records (including the right to access them) and required the U.S. Department of Health and Human Services (DHHS) to develop regulations protecting the privacy and security of health information held in either paper or digital form.*

◊   *In 2009 DHHS released a final rule under HIPAA mandating that all providers covered by HIPAA implement ICD-10 for medical coding when submitting bills to any payer. The final deadline for adoption of ICD-10 was October 1, 2015. There were incentives for early compliance, and a serious penalty for failure to comply in that, after the deadline, payers could reject any claims not submitted with ICD-10 coding.*

◊   *Title IV of the 2009 American Recovery and Reinvestment Act (Recovery Act) called for the universal adoption of EHRs capable of being shared across The Provider Universe, as well as with patients. The Recovery Act stipulated a deadline of January 1, 2015, for meaningful-use compliance and provided incentives for early compliance and penalties for failure to meet the deadline.*

◊   *The Patient Protection and Affordable Care Act of 2010 (Affordable Care Act or 2010 ACA - Popular Nickname: Obamacare) went beyond insurance to address the need for long-term changes in health-care quality, the organization and design of health-care delivery, and HIT transparency. It laid the foundation for system-wide performance reporting that will enable patients to get up-to-date information regarding their own health care, as well as the performance of their health-care providers.*

◊   *Medicare Access and CHIP Reauthorization Act of 2015 (MACRA), effective January 1, 2017, which incentivizes physicians to move from fee-for-service to value-based payment, aka pay-for-performance, requires that qualifying physicians acquire and submit in digital form data relating to key areas of quality and cost measurement, as well as progress toward meaningful use of digital technology.*

Enforcement of legislation was deemed the responsibility of the DHHS, particularly the Office for Civil Rights (OCR) and the Centers for Medicare & Medicaid Services (CMS), the largest payer of health-care claims in the country. Clearly, policymakers were serious about first encouraging and then requiring providers to go digital in the pursuit of improving care quality and controlling costs.

This meant that what had been a somewhat random, generally voluntary progress toward (1) improving information quality through up-to-date coding and (2) the digitization of health records became a requirement capable of interrupting provider income flow if not met. And meeting that requirement proved to be a challenge. Not only was massive change required as to billing and record-keeping, but intensified hacking activity made cybersecurity an increasingly serious issue.

For providers, the key aspects of the HIT challenge are:

◊ **ICD-10** —*The most-recent version of the International Classification of Diseases, a reporting format issued in 1999 by the World Health Organization (WHO) to standardize the collection, reporting, and other uses of mortality statistics around the world. Although ICD is based on mortality, its primary use is to identify specific health issues. That is, via the use of 68,000 codes, ICD-10 "slices and dices" causes of death to reflect the current understanding of medical conditions, diagnoses, and outcomes. The result is that ICD enables the sharing of specific diagnoses and best practices in treatment in a format instantly understandable wherever it is used. ICD-10 improved preceding versions by (1) allowing for more detail and specificity in the code set, (2) modernizing terminology and making codes more consistent throughout, and (3) setting forth combinations of diagnoses and symptoms, thereby simplifying the reporting of complex conditions. ICD-10 not only improves the accuracy of information shared among providers, but is also required for billing. Beginning October, 1, 2015, health-care bills submitted to any payer must employ ICD-10 codes.*

◊ **Electronic health records (EHRs)** — *records of a patient's care and related information held and shared in a digital format accessible to the patient and the patient's care team. The purpose of the records is to (1) avoid duplicative treatment, (2) reduce errors, (3) increase patient engagement in self-management of health care, (4) make it possible to share, in a private, secure manner, accurate, consistent information relating to patients and their care with all those having a need and right to know, (5) improve public health by better communication between public-health agencies and providers and by* *pinpointing disparities in health in the general population, (6) protect HIT from hacking, and (7) decrease the possibility of fraud against payers. The deadline for providers to prove "meaningful use" of EHRs was January 1, 2015.*

◊ **Computerized Provider Order Entry (CPOE)** — *requirement that physicians make computer entry of all information and orders relating to patients. CPOE represents a major change in the recording of patient histories, keeping of diagnostic and treatment records, and the ordering process relating to patient care, including medication pre-scriptions. CPOE is an essential part of the move to EHRs.*

◊ **Clinical Decision Support System (CDSS)** — *software that gives physicians and their staffs access to a database of latest discoveries, diag-nostics, best practices, clinical trials, and outcomes relating to a patient's specific condition. New care-delivery models assume that physicians will employ CDSS and will share the information with patients and their families, when appropriate, as part of the process that develops a treatment plan. Used correctly, CDSS is supposed to improve diagnosis and treatment quality, reduce errors, and reduce costs.*

◊ **MACRA** — *2015 program that incentivizes physicians to move from fee-for-service to value-based payment, aka pay-for-performance. MACRA requires that independent physicians report data relating to (1) quality of care, (2) resource use (i.e., cost-effectiveness), (3) clinical practice improvement activities, and (4) meaningful use of certified EHR technology.*

◊ **HIT Security** — *recognized as a critical issue as early as the 1996 HIPAA legislation. Providers, especially hospitals, and insurance plans are attractive targets for hackers because of (1) the value of the infor-mation contained in their digital records, making them salable on the Dark Web or usable for purposes of blackmail and (2) the fact that at least some providers have been known to pay ransom to get hacker-en-crypted systems back online. Providers and payers are vulnerable to hacking because of (1) the large number of potential users with a right or need to access patient and other information, often from private devices; with inadequate security; (2) the need for provider and payer HIT to remain operative 24/7 in order to maintain critical services and processes; (3) outdated or inadequate firewalls and virus-detec-tion on hospital or physician-office servers, as well as those of at least some payers; (4) the need for up-to-date training for IT managers that* *focuses on security; and (5) the growing sophistication of hackers.*

A mini-industry sprang up to support the transition to ICD-10 and EHRs, to simplify data collection and reporting as per MACRA, and to improve cyber-security. The last is a particular concern for large and teaching hospitals, which according to an April 2017 research report in the *Journal of the American Medical Association (JAMA)* are at particular risk of data breaches. In 2016 alone 1,798 hospital breaches are estimated to have occurred, with more than a third affecting either large hospitals or academic medical centers.

Significance For The Provider Universe

Providers had to come to terms quickly with various kinds of IT consultants, complex software that had to be either purchased or accessed via subscription, the need to update computer systems and to train staff to use the new software and equipment, and maintenance of the new systems.

In addition to these considerations was the loss of time as staff got up to speed with the coding and recordkeeping requirements. All of this together rep-resented a significant investment by providers, which was probably why their professional associations by and large resisted the requirements. CMS held firm, however, deeming the move to digitization and up-to-date coding essential.

Even providers with IT staffs have found it hard to keep up with HIT man-dates. As for others, especially smaller physician practices, compliance has been anywhere from frustrating to nightmarish. For all providers, compliance has required huge amounts of resource.

It would be difficult to overstate the importance of getting HIT right. Patients who share (or allow to be shared) sensitive information put not only their lives but also their financial health in the hands of provider and payer processes. The ability of The Provider Universe to use HIT to benefit patients and not harm them is a credibility issue, as is its ability to bill payers quickly and accurately.

The Bottom Line

Getting HIT right is an issue not only of credibility but of integrity, for the records are where the line gets drawn in the sand for The Provider Universe, the payers that support it, and the patients who enter it. Unfortunately, "right" is easier said than done. Dealing with HIT issues — especially cybersecurity — is like the expe-rience of the little Dutch boy with his finger in the dike: the water rises constantly and the tide continues to come in.

Chapter Fifteen.

Major Challenge: Emerging Care-Delivery Models & Reimbursement

The Provider Universe has relatively recently had to cope with several major changes in care delivery and reimbursement that have the power to transform traditional medicine.

Summary Of Issues Related To Emerging Care-Delivery Models & Reimbursement

Until recently, care-delivery models changed little in the last century from the perspective of either provider or patient. Care was delivered with a tight focus, with each provider treating an intervention relating to a particular health issue as a one-off event. There was no systematic consideration as to outcomes, quality of care, continuity of care, or cost-effectiveness of care.

Traditionally, billing for each intervention was on a fee-for-service basis, submitted by each provider separately, and charges were often shown as *X amount for visit of whatever date*, with only a final amount or brief summary of charges indicated. Outcomes or the concept of best practices did not enter into billing. Nor did they enter into payment — if the payer accepted the charge as legitimate, whether as billed or negotiated downwards, payment was made in full within a normal business turnaround time frame.

In recent decades, the billing process has changed. All charges have been coded; and billing has been generally "unbundled," that is each part of each service is billed and/or broken out separately by each of the providers involved. This has led to duplicative billing and other errors and coincided with an explosion in health-care costs.

Clearly, things had to change, for the trend of exploding costs could not be sustained when the huge cohort of Baby Boomers reached the age of Medicare eligibility, which was also the age their health-care needs would increase. The initial response was legislation and regulation that attempted, with only limited success, to control costs arbitrarily by tying them to general economic indicators. Complicating the situation was the parallel effort to improve care outcomes.

Recent legislation has gone much further, mandating that Medicare aid and incentivize experimentation in care-delivery and reimbursement. Since 2010 this has seen the ACA's Center for Medicare and Medicaid Innovation (CMMI or CMS Innovation Center) drive innovation by means of demonstration projects with 61,000 providers that it has run, financed, or partnered with states to implement.

Some of these delivery experiments simply modify existing provider methods to make them more effective. Others test the expansion of services, such as doctor house calls. Others focus on how reimbursement to providers is handled. This often involves a combination of fee-for-service and capitation and sees providers being allowed a set dollar amount per patient on top of their regular fees, allowing them to spend more time with patients on preventive care, hire extra staff to improve service, or experiment with telemedicine – all of which should improve care and lower costs.

Thousands of experiments are being tried via CMMI, and those that meet the dual criteria of improving quality and cutting costs will be scaled up.

The two delivery models that at this point are the "stars" of delivery innovation are (1) Accountable Care Organizations (ACOs) and (2) Patient-Centered Medical Homes (PCMHs). These models, known as APMs (alternate payment models) affect not only how care is delivered but also how it is billed and reimbursed. APMs move away from fee-for-service and unbundled billing and toward value-based (pay-for performance), bundled billing.

In ACOs, all providers involved in a defined health episode or period of care bill as part of a team, usually with a hospital or physician as the primary billing contact for the payer. Ideally, charges are to be bundled, that is, submitted as a group in a total amount with supporting codes. Payer reimbursement is risk-based, that is, not everything billed will necessarily be paid, as a portion of the reimbursement is tied to quality of outcomes and cost-effectiveness. The ACO contract agreed to by the team determines how the resulting reimbursement is to be distributed. It is the team collectively, not its individual members, that the payer assesses on quality of care and cost-effectiveness. Payer reimbursement is made in two stages, with a predetermined percentage being paid within normal turnaround, while the remainder is retained for a set period of time until outcomes and cost-effectiveness can be determined. The determination relies in part on comparative metrics from other providers. ACOs producing high-quality outcomes in a cost-effective manner will be paid all of the percentage retained (and may also earn bonuses). ACOs producing less-than-satisfactory metrics on these elements will be paid only a portion of the amount retained, or perhaps none of it.

In essence, the ACO arrangement gives the entire billing group the incentive to work together to plan and execute the care most likely to produce the best result in terms of both patient outcome and cost. It gives individual members of the group the incentive to deliver what is required to support the group's strategy in that, if they do not, other members will not want to incorporate them in future ACO groups. According to "Accountable Care Organizations in 2016: Private And Public-Sector Growth And Dispersion" in the HealthAffairs Blog of April 21, 2016, the concept continues to grow in popularity, albeit to different degrees in different states, with California, Florida, Illinois, New York, Massachusetts, Pennsylvania, and Texas in the lead. Leavitt Partners, in conjunction with the Accountable Care Learning Collaborative, says that as of the end of January 2016 there were 838 active ACOs covering 28.3 million people.

The PCMH (Patient-Centered Medical Home) represents a basic rethinking of how primary care is organized and delivered. Here, the focus is not on individual care episodes or a limited amount of time but more on lifelong patient health. The individual provider becomes part of a team — including hospitals, physicians (MDs), nurse practitioners (NPs), advanced-practice nurses (APRNs), physician assistants (PAs), registered nurses (RNs), licensed practical nurses (LPNs), pharmacists, nutritionists, social workers, coordinators, and any other entities involved — who are jointly responsible for a patient's ongoing comprehensive care. This includes prevention and wellness, acute care, and chronic care, whether physical and/or mental. This patient-centered approach requires strong relationship building among providers and between providers and patient. This approach makes it possible for the PCMH team to provide care that relates not just to a specific medical condition or episode but also to the patient's medical history, cultural background, values, and preferences. Inevitably, this means patients must become partners in their own care, helping the members of the health-care team to develop treatment plans that will work for them. Facilitating patient involvement is the requirement that a member of the PCMH team be available to patients 24/7 via email or phone. Providers involved in a PCMH bill their services individually, using bundled billing.

According to the Patient-Centered Primary Care Collaborative, there are approximately 500 public and private sector PCMH initiatives being tracked across the U.S. Primary Care Progress reports that, overall, patients, payers, and providers are increasingly pleased with PCMH outcomes.

Providers in both ACO and PCMH alternate payment models have a big incentive to persuade patients to do a better job of self-management as to health. No matter how technically successful a medical intervention, a patient who fails to undergo the full course of recommended treatment and/or to follow doctor's orders as to medication, diet, exercise, etc., is more likely to have a poor outcome. This is not only unfortunate for the patient, but affects the reimbursement the provider(s) will be allowed under pay-for-performance guidelines.

An interesting twist to care delivery relates to the ability of insurance plans to limit patient choices of providers through narrow networks or even capitation. Increasingly, as insurance-company competition declines due to mergers, the networks tend to narrow, limited to those providers willing to accept highly competitive rates for services. Providers that refuse the rates offered by the insurance company are eliminated from the company's network, thus (1) forcing that provider's patients covered under company plans to seek care elsewhere and (2) decreasing provider income literally overnight. When the insurance company adopts a capitation model, customer choice as to providers becomes even more narrow because each customer in a geographic area is assigned to a specific provider for specific services. In capitation agreements, in each designated period, the insurance company pays the provider a set amount for each enrolled person assigned to it. The provider is paid this money (1) whether or not the enrollee uses medical care during the period and (2) whatever the quantity or value of the service provided.

Significance For The Provider Universe

Different parts of provider operations are affected by these emerging care-delivery and reimbursement trends, but there is also a collective significance.

◊　*Provider authority over payers and patients has been significantly eroded.*

◊　*Provider revenue stream is less predictable as to both amount and timing.*

◊　*Provider independence is at least psychologically curtailed by the need to negotiate with patients, payers, and other providers.*

◊　*Provider performance is being influenced by (1) access to decision-support tools and (2) comparisons with other providers.*

◊　*Patients are more questioning of provider recommendations and potentially less loyal to any particular provider.*

Perhaps the development arising from changes in care delivery and reimbursement that holds the greatest potential for a higher quality, more cost-effective future for health care lies in the fact that patients will be increasingly better informed about health, care, and the truth that "the silver bullet" cannot be counted on to vanquish unhealthy lifestyle choices and habits.

The Bottom Line

The Provider Universe was once an opaque place that held its mysteries close to its well-protected chest. Unless they were willing to spend a lot of time in the library, all patients could learn about their ailments was what their doctors chose to tell them. As for talking about charges, many doctors (and their staffs) would have considered that beyond the pale. Patients who wanted to know what was involved in making care decisions were usually seen as "buttinskys" and potential troublemakers. No one on the provider or payer end was particularly interested in patients doing anything other than (1) following doctor's orders and (2) paying their health-insurance premiums on time.

To say, yet again, that times have changed is to point out the obvious.

Changes in care delivery and reimbursement are in the process of creating a very different environment, one that is more transparent as to activities, outcomes, and charges. This is also an environment in which it becomes increasingly difficult for providers to anticipate revenue streams. This last factor alone favors larger, better-capitalized providers.

Chapter Sixteen.

Major Challenge: Patient Empowerment

The concept of patient empowerment is a relatively recent development in The Provider Universe. In the past, patients were expected to be generally passive consumers of health care. They delivered their symptoms, were told what to do, said thank you, paid the bill, and went home or to another provider, where the process was repeated.

The only recourse patients had when they felt they had received inadequate health care was to report the provider to whichever state agency regulated providers and/or to any professional associations that kept track of such complaints. Apart from this, they had few legal rights other than not to be treated with such obvious ineptitude that they had grounds for a lawsuit. They didn't even have the automatic right to access their health-care records. In fact, prior to 1996, patient rights to health information was determined state by state, and access was often severely restricted.

Summary of Issues Relating to Patient Empowerment

Empowerment of patients is both formal and informal, and derives from legislation, regulation, and Internet access.

Formal, nationwide patient empowerment began with COBRA (Consolidated Omnibus Budget Reconciliation Act), the 1986 federal legislation that gave workers who lose their group health benefits the right to continue those benefits for a set period by assuming personal responsibility for premium payment. COBRA was important because, at the least, it allowed individuals time to make other arrangements before being excluded from the employer's group plan. In worst-case scenarios, it enabled employees to keep insurance they might not otherwise be able to obtain at once due to ongoing health issues.

In 1996, HIPAA gave patients nationwide wide-ranging rights over their medical information and what could be done with it. Those rights included not only privacy and security of health records, but also patient access. For the first time, as the DHHS puts it, Americans had "a legal, enforceable right to see and receive copies upon request of the information in their medical and other health records maintained by their health care providers and health plans."

The result of the 1996 Act was that patients could request copies of their records from providers and insurance plans. While the federal law gave patients this basic right, state laws could modify the exact process the patient must follow. Also, some providers and payers had their own variations on what was required for access.

When combined with the mandated move to electronic health records (EHRs — see **Chapter Fourteen.** *Major Challenge: Information Technology*), this means that, for the first time in history — once all providers are in full compliance with EHR provisions and patient access has been set up (both of which elements are still being implemented across The Provider Universe as of 2017) — patients should have fast, easy, secure access to all their medical records. This will allow patients to acquire knowledge that will make it possible for them "to be more in control of decisions regarding their health and well-being." Patients may also continue to request their records in non-electronic formats, such as paper copies or faxes, for which there may or may not be a charge.

A simultaneously occurring initiative propelled by the 2010 ACA — the move to the PCMH (Patient-Centered Medical Home) — accelerates patient empowerment. A core concept of PCMH is that providers fully involve patients (and, when appropriate, their families) in the health-care process. In PCMH, it becomes the responsibility of providers to consider patients within the context of their personal circumstances and to respect patient beliefs and preferences as to treatment. A basic requirement is patient access to records, as well as 24/7 access by either phone or email to a PCMH representative.

One of the most-important provisions of the 2010 ACA made it illegal for insurance companies to use preexisting conditions as a reason to deny or limit coverage. This change gave patients a significant advantage in deciding when to obtain health insurance, even as it removed one of the primary techniques employed by health insurers to maintain higher profits by not insuring individuals who were already known to be in likely need of medial care.

Perhaps the major form of patient empowerment is self-directed and is made possible by the Internet. Individuals can, thanks to increasingly targeted search engines, research just about anything relating to health care; and many do. Patients can do more than research, however. Those who are so inclined can read and leave reviews for their providers on a wide range of ranking sites.

Also important are the patient-satisfaction surveys sent by payers and providers following certain kinds of care episodes. The way in which patients complete these forms can have a significant impact on provider reimbursement.

Perhaps the most official-sounding part of patient empowerment is *informed consent*. This is permission given by a patient — or an authorized representative acting on his or her behalf — for health-care intervention to be performed on a patient's person. Guidelines for the wording and method of informed consent, as well as how the provider gets it from the patient, are based on medical ethics and/or research ethics, depending on the kind of intervention that is proposed. Theoretically, informed consent is deemed to have been given when a provider explains to the patient the purpose and implications of the proposed intervention — that is, its purpose, risks, and likely outcome — in a way that is clearly understood by the patient who then agrees either orally or in writing to the intervention. That is not as simple as it sounds. Providers are not always totally candid about the full range of risks an intervention involves. Patients who appear to be listening may just be pretending. Patients who appear to understand may not always. Patients rarely ask questions; and, when they do, experience suggests that providers often act impatient or hurried as if the patient is inconveniencing them by requiring what the provider considers unnecessary time out of a busy day. Oftentimes, from the time-pressured provider's perspective, informed consent is frequently more about CYA for legal reasons than it is that patients actually be informed. At the same time, despite its imperfections, the very existence of the requirement for informed consent gives patients power they did not have before it was required, even if they don't always choose to use it or providers make it implicitly difficult to use.

Combined with other legal protections for patients, informed consent is a potent enabler of patient empowerment.

Another powerful enabler is the 1998 Consumer Bill of Rights and Responsibilities, issued by the Advisory Commission on Consumer Protection and Quality in the Health Care Industry. This Bill of Rights, developed by the federal government, is used not only by government-sponsored health plans but by various private plans. Because of it, providers understand that patients have the right to:

◊ *Information disclosure adequate to support informed health-care decisions*

◊ *Choice of providers, within the patient's health plan*

◊ *Access to emergency services when needed*

◊ *Participation in treatment decisions, including the right to know all treatment options even if not covered by the patient's health plan*

◊ *Respect and nondiscrimination while seeking and undergoing health care*

◊ *Confidentiality of health information*

◊ *Access to their health-care records*

◊ *A "fair, fast, and objective" review of any complaints against health plans, doctors, hospitals, or other health-care personnel*

Ultimately, patient empowerment represents an extension of the American consumer movement into health care, demanding that the industry treat the individuals who purchase its expensive services as customers as well as patients.

The flip side of the 1998 Consumer Bill of Rights and Responsibilities is the second "R" – "Responsibilities." The stipulations are both basic and far-reaching, calling for patients to assume accountability for self-management of care (including healthy habits and the avoidance of spreading disease), to be truthful in the information given providers, to work with providers to get the best diagnosis and treatment plan and then to follow it, to recognize the limits and risks of medicine, to know insurance-plan provisions, to pay medical bills, and to report health-care wrongdoing and fraud to the appropriate authorities.

While the 1998 document is not itself law, CMS and various insurance companies accept it as appropriate guidance for both consumers and providers, and the concept is incorporated in certain legislation. Many consumers are glad to accept the benefits of the "Rights" but don't appear to have grasped the need to pay more attention to the "Responsibilities." Given the growing impact that patient outcomes will have on provider income under new reimbursement models, it isn't unreasonable to suspect that (1) some providers may begin to winnow from their patient lists those individuals who ignore their responsibilities in a way that undermines a good outcome and (2) some insurance plans may begin to balk at paying for treatment made necessary only by poor consumer habits.

Significance For The Provider Universe

Patient empowerment signals a basic shift in the balance of power between patients, providers, and payers.

◊ *Whatever their ethnicity or occupation, individuals can obtain health insurance even if they are ill and/or older.*

◊ *Individuals have the right to access their health records, which should increasingly incorporate their full health history and not simply that related to a specific event.*

◊ *Individuals have certain rights over what providers and payers do with their health information.*

◊ *Patients being treated for any medical condition have the right to be given information by their providers that helps them make informed decisions as to their health care. Providers must respect a patient's decision even if they don't agree with it.*

◊ *Patients whose care is provided within a PCMH arrangement have the right to expect that (1) they will be consulted as to treatment plans and (2) all providers in their health-care "community" are working with other providers to address the totality of their health needs.*

◊   *Providers in a PCMH must be prepared to spend more time with patients and other providers in the patient's care chain — sharing information, answering questions, and seeking input.*

◊   *Providers are more likely to be confronted by patients bearing printouts of information from the Internet, information that will have influenced patient attitudes toward a health event before the provider has a chance to examine the patient and offer his or her diagnosis and treatment plan.*

◊   *Patients can leave ratings online, thus influencing other patients in their choice of providers.*

◊   *Patients can complete patient-satisfaction surveys as to the care they receive from providers, thus influencing provider reimbursement.*

◊   *Patients have a wider range of choices for certain kinds of care and can readily get information as to their comparative merits.*

◊   *Patients have both legally enforceable rights, as well as what might be called "rights by custom," but may also become subject to assessment as to their efforts to fulfill their responsibilities in regard to their care.*

Patient empowerment, then, is overall an excellent step forward in giving us a more-significant voice in our care. At the same time, it's related to growing expectations of how much individual responsibility we are prepared to assume for helping providers to produce good patient outcomes.

The Bottom Line

The appearance of patient empowerment as a permanent goal of payers will accelerate competition within The Provider Universe, pressure providers to get EHRs set up as quickly as possible, give patients more control over how health issues are treated, and accelerate a trend toward demanding greater accountability from providers as to outcome and patients as to lifestyle choices and health-affecting habits. Patients will be expected by both providers and payers to take a more-active, positive role in the health-care process by following doctor's orders and also by taking better care of themselves. Moreover, behavior monitors or implanted sensing devices will give payers and providers information as to patient habits. Ultimately, rather than risk nonpayment due to outcomes, providers may choose not to treat patients who repeatedly ignore treatment plans, withhold information necessary to provide "best practices" care, and/or refuse to pay bills.

Chapter Seventeen.

Major Challenge: The Political-Football Factor

Health care has gone from being a "home and hearth" issue to one capable of generating extreme political reactions across the entire population, reactions that make coherent policy formulation extremely difficult. In large part, this is because:

> ◊ *Over time, American health care has evolved into a vast Rubik's Cube made up of public programs and private enterprise so interlocked as to make adjusting any one part likely to upend another segment that, at first glance, appears to have no connection.*

> ◊ *The need to address the health-care issue confronts all concerned with an almost perfect example of ideology at war with logistical reality.*

Also, the issue affords politicians of the purely self-serving variety the opportunity to "score points" by grandstanding, pronouncing whatever they think will gain them the greatest advantage at a given moment. Also, so much money is involved that associations of insurance companies and providers automatically gird themselves for however big a fight they feel is necessary to protect their interests.

Summary Of Issues Relating To The Political-Football Factor

Issues arise from the contradictions caused by the efforts of lobbyists, the influence of political contributors, the ideological orientation of legislators, and the inconsistent attitudes of the general citizenry as to the proper role of government in health care.

As mentioned in **Chapter Six:** *Who Regulates, Influences, And Legislates Various Aspects of Health Care?*, lobbyists represent (1) every segment of The Provider Universe and their related associations, (2) the payers who support The Provider Universe, (3) non-health associations or other entities that do not want government money spent on health that could, they feel, be better spent on their industry, and (4) ideologically based organizations that want more or less government involvement in health care according to their beliefs as to the proper role of government. The aim of lobbyists is to convince legislators that the association, industry, or company they represent is worthy of whatever attention it is that they want at the moment — passage of a law, repeal of a law, change in regulation, whatever. Lobbyists exert influence by personal contact and discussions with elected and appointed officials and their staffs, during which they share the perspective of the entity that employs them. These contacts often involve providing politicians with materials that will assist them in their governmental role, including position papers and detailed statistical analyses relating to the lobbyists' issues. Sometimes, this can also involve lobbyist-paid junkets to appealing locales to "study the issues."

Political contributors influence politicians by increasing or decreasing the amounts of money they give to a politician's campaign, the increase or decrease usually being tied to the degree to which the politician supports the contributor's position on key issues.

The amount of influence that contributors and lobbyists have on elected and appointed officials relates to some extent to the individual official's political ideology. An official who shares the basic mindset of those attempting to influence her or him is more likely to listen receptively to what it is that the lobbyist or contributor wants done or undone.

As this isn't meant to be a comprehensive analysis of a complex topic, it's probably enough to say that, insofar as ideology affects health-care policy, there are essentially four broad schools of thought in the U.S., listed below in order from those advocating the least government involvement to those advocating the most.

◊ **PURE FREE-MARKET** — *Government at any level should play no role in health care, which should be provided within an environment controlled only by market forces without any government oversight or intervention. Government should not have health programs like Medicare and Medicaid. Individuals should have the right to buy health insurance from private businesses without any sort of government interference, subsidy, or support other than government enforcement of contracts entered into between private businesses and individuals. Individuals should have the right to choose whichever provider they want and receive care without government interference or oversight of quality, safety, or cost. Government should not vet the safety of health products or the accuracy of advertising for health products or services, including health insurance. Nor should government review insurance policies for premium consistency and clarity of wording. Nor should government have the right to inspect the premises of health-care providers for hygiene purposes, nor control the number or size of hospitals that can be built, nor pass laws protecting the safety* or health of personnel who work in them or patients who use them. Nor should government subsidize medical research, the teaching of medicine, the testing of procedures, the licensing of health professionals, or anything else to do with ensuring the safety, cost, and effectiveness of health care, thus making health care a matter of ongoing negotiation between individuals and business. In this pure free-market approach, health care is treated like a commercial commodity, patients are consumers, and there are no consumer protections. The basic assumption is that: (1) government at every level is inherently inefficient and/or corrupt and cannot be trusted to use resources properly to benefit citizens; (2) individual health or access to care is in no way and to no degree the responsibility of government at any level; (3) providers and insurance plans will be motivated to provide the best care and service because they are competing for customers; and (4) customers will acquire the information necessary to make choices that will benefit their health interests and, if not, it is their problem and not that of the state.

◊ **CURRENT SYSTEM BUT WITH MODIFICATIONS THAT PRIVATIZE SIGNIFICANT SEGMENTS** — *Government should play a major role in health care in that it continues to ensure the safety, quality, and effectiveness of care, but certain medical programs that are now the province of government should be privatized, particularly programs like Medicare that act to insure participants against costs. Government would still underwrite costs in the form of vouchers and other subsidies, but individuals would have no guarantees as to coverage but simply the right to enter the commercial health-care insurance marketplace and use those vouchers or subsidies to purchase some form of care that might or might not be the equivalent of what they had under the terminated government program. In this modified free-market approach, health care is treated like a qualified right and a government-subsidized commercial commodity, patients are consumers who remain responsible for certain costs but who are protected from potentially negative consequences of misprepresentation as to quality and safety of products and services, and there are limited consumer protections. The basic assumption is that: (1) government should regulate safety and quality of care; (2) private insurers can do a better, more cost-effective job of paying for health care than government, thus containing costs; and (3) government has the responsibility of ensuring that private insurers do not lose money by assuming what was previously a function of government.*

◊ **CURRENT SYSTEM BUT WITH MODIFICATIONS THAT IMPROVE ACCESS, QUALITY, AND SAFETY** — *Government should remain fully involved in ensuring the safety, quality, and accessibility of health care. Health care would remain essentially private, but government would incentivize reform in certain aspects of the health-care industry to make it deliver better outcomes, be more cost-effective, and improve accessibility to qualified U.S. residents. Reform would pay particular attention to care-delivery models, billing methods, prevention, and public-health issues. In this model, health care is treated like a qualified right, patients are clients who remain responsible for certain costs, and there is significant ongoing government effort in making sure that both payers (government programs, insurance companies, and employers self-insured as to employee health care) and clients get their money's worth. The basic assumption is that: (1) government has a legitimate role to play in maintaining quality, controlling costs, and coordinating the transformation of today's health care into that rapidly being made possible by technological improvements and advances; (2) health care should remain essentially a private enterprise and private insurance plans have an important role to play; and (3) it is appropriate for government to subsidize private insurance plans if this is necessary to ensure their continued viability.*

◊ **SINGLE-PAYER, UNIVERSAL HEALTH CARE** — *Government should assume the responsibility for health care for anyone resident in the U.S., whether citizens or not, whether here legally or not. Government would play an expanded role in prevention and there would be public clinics and hospitals. A private health industry would continue to exist that would be regulated as to safety and effectiveness, but government would assume payment of costs and set the criteria for how health-care providers would be paid. Individuals would have the right not only to treatment of existing medical conditions, but also to preventive care. There would be no deductibles, co-pays, or other out-of-pocket expenses for users of health-care services. The details of an ideal single-payer, universal health-care system as it would be applied in the U.S. — particularly as to the role of commercial and employer insurance plans — are somewhat fuzzy, but they would probably resemble those in other industrialized nations (the U.S. is the only industrialized nation in the world without a national health system). In the national-health systems of other industrialized nations, there is significant correlation between public health and individual health. In this single-payer, universal health-care model, health care (including* *prevention) is treated like a basic human right, patients are clients, and no one resident in the U.S. would be denied free health care. The basic assumption is that government responsibility to protect citizens and other residents incorporates the responsibility to protect them from the consequences of ill health or injury.*

Elected and appointed officials — like the rest of us — are rarely 100% consistent. Individually, in fact, it's likely that their personal beliefs incline them toward a combination of elements from more than one of the above. Politicians, however, tend to hew to the stated policies of the party under whose banner they campaigned and were elected. Even there, however, there is a certain amount of wiggle room. This wiggle room is made up not only of inconsistencies in the individual politician's belief system but also in his or her need to remain appealing to the electorate that voted for her or him and to have the organizational and financial support of powerful entities, like major industries and influential associations. It is in this wiggle-room area that lobbyists and political contributors operate in order to get the best return for their efforts and money.

The final factor in creating the "political football" atmosphere in which American health care now exists is us, the people who must use the system to stay well or get well. As with the other factors described above, we each have an individual perspective on what health care should involve, including who should provide it and where, how much it should be regulated, what it should cost, and who should pay for it. There are so many perspectives, in fact, and they involve so much cross-hatching of needs, preferences, and ideologies that summarization is hard. Probably the most definitive thing that can be said is that we tend to think in terms of "us" vs. "them", with "them" being anyone other than "us", for example:

◊   *The care "we" need or want is appropriate and that needed or wanted by "them" may be disproportionate.*

◊   *"We" deserve health care while "they" may not.*

◊   *If ill or injured, "we" should have access to whatever remedy has even the slightest chance of curing us, whatever the cost, but "they" should be content with remedies proven to be both generally successful and cost-effective.*

◊   *It is perfectly acceptable for government and employer-sponsored health plans to provide or pay for "our" care but unreasonable for "them" to expect this same degree of support.*

Also, like legislators, we are all over the place ideologically speaking, but our ideology, like theirs, is not necessarily consistent. Generally, if a health-care policy obviously benefits us, we view it as necessary and justifiable; and if its benefits to us are less-obvious or nonexistent, we view it as superfluous and indefensible.

Significance For The Provider Universe

All the interests that compete for ascendancy in the political decision-making process as it relates to health care are in what amounts to an ongoing war for points made and ground gained in enemy territory. Lobbyists justify their continued employment by demonstrating to clients their clout with legislators — bills passed or repealed, issues highlighted or neutralized, alliances formed or dissolved, etc. Political contributors, many also the funders of lobbying efforts, donate money to campaigns of legislators who "vote their way" on health issues. Legislators tend to follow the direct or implied dictates of well-connected lobbyists and well-heeled political contributors, as well as the official policy of the party to which they belong — at least until it becomes clear that doing so will imperil their chances of being reelected when those dictates become known and are obviously against the interests of their constituents.

The on-the-ground, practical result of all of this for providers includes: (1) continually shifting priorities; (2) wildly fluctuating income projections; and (3) unpredictable time frames for reimbursement.

All this leaves providers in an odd position. Through their industry or professional associations, they are themselves political contributors and major funders of lobbying efforts, and so they exert a certain degree of influence on legislation and regulation. At the same time, many politicians appear indifferent to or ignorant of the need for provider stability and continuity; and political grandstanding to make points with lobbyists, contributors, and/or constituents can have a devastating effect on provider outlook and viability.

Perhaps the most outstanding example of a manifestation of this kind of problem is when legislators pass a law, call it *Law B,* that provides support for certain kinds of medical services, thereby ending a different form of support stipulated in *Law A,* then later repeal *Law B* without reinstating *Law A* or making any other provision for the now-missing support. Another example of the lack of political forethought as to the impact of legislation and regulation is the tendency of new heads of agencies charged with oversight or facilitation of provider priorities to arrive with a "not invented here" mindset. In other words, if the incoming head didn't think of the innovation, it is automatically questionable and subject to massive change.

That wouldn't be so troubling if medical practices and hospitals didn't spend years preparing to deliver care by certain methods or to bill in a certain way, investing significant amounts of money and time to conform to their understanding of current requirements, only to have a "new broom" sweep away much of what the providers are set up to support.

The Bottom Line

It's ultimately legislators and those whose appointments they influence or control who shape legislation and regulation affecting health care in the U.S. Legislative action is shaped by (1) the interests of lobbyists and political contributors, (2) the attitudes of constituents, (3) ideological beliefs on the part of politicians, and (4) official policy of the party to which the politician belongs. Unfortunately, if there is a moral high ground in health-care policy that fairly balances patient needs, provider priorities, and payer viability, it has so far been impossible to find.

Chapter Eighteen.

Physicians Caught In A Perfect Storm

All parts of The Provider Universe are affected by the major challenges of medical advances and new technology, information technology, emerging care-delivery models, reimbursement changes, patient empowerment, and politics. It's unlikely, however, that any part of the health-care system is experiencing more pressure from these and other factors than physicians, the profession with which medicine is most identified.

There are several kinds of physicians: primary care; specialist; surgeon; and dentist. Traditionally, it is physicians who "call the shots" in U.S. health care, who use their training, experience, intelligence, and intuition to perform the most-critical medical functions: diagnosis; surgery; and medication prescription. Their professional association, the American Medical Association (AMA), is the most-powerful health-care organization in the U.S. and one of the two or three most powerful in any industry, with a major political presence in the form of lobbying and campaign contributions.

The reader wishing to understand the "how" and "why" of twenty-first century American health care must take a closer look at what is happening with physicians, in particular primary-care physicians, for it is in their offices most Americans first come into contact with the health-care system. Further, it is their assessments and diagnoses that start patients on the path that most of them will subsequently follow as they move through The Provider Universe. This gives the primary-care physician a degree of influence unmatched by any other provider. The changes now roiling their once-peaceful environments have a profound effect on patient care.

Yesterday's Physicians: The Way They Were

Historically, primary-care physicians and even most specialists had solo practices or worked in small physician-owned practices with ten or fewer physicians with similar or complementary specialties. The practices were generally set up as sole proprietorships or partnerships. In this setting, physicians enjoyed the advantages of autonomy. Their own boss, they were in control of the shape and evolution of the practice, focused on medical care, and had a staff small enough and a patient base stable enough to enable them to develop close, personal relationships with both employees and patients. In this setting, physicians can, as the American College of Physicians (ACP) puts it, "provide your own unique style of medical care."

Today's Physicians: Changing Times

In the more-complicated environment that has emerged in the last three decades, physician autonomy has been eroded by a wide range of ongoing, disruptive issues, including:

◊   *Medical-school debt burden*

◊   *Cost of doing business*

◊   *Career path: Employee vs. independent practitioner*

◊   *Emerging practice models*

◊   *Growing importance of nonclinical support-staff specialties*

◊   *Payment issues*

◊   *MACRA and Medicare payment reform*

◊   *2010 Patient Protection and Affordable Care Act*

◊   *The elephant in the room: Medicare*

◊   *Health-insurance company consolidation*

◊   *Complementary and competitive occupations*

◊   *Increasing competition*

◊   *When the practice of medicine became a trade*

◊   *Shortage of physicians*

◊   *Less pressure and greater mobility - at a price*

◊   *Unending advances in medical knowledge and new technologies*

◊   *Board certification*

◊   *Change in professional status*

For physicians in private practice — most of whom were drawn to medicine by intellectual challenge, the prestige the role confers, income potential, and/or the value of the profession to those it serves — these issues erode morale and undermine confidence. Even so, they suggest the new reality that all physicians, whether primary-care or specialist, must now navigate or risk the loss of much toward which they have worked.

Medical School Debt Burden

Doctors whose parents didn't pay for medical school and who did not receive other assistance typically start their careers with significant debt — over $180,000 on average according to the Association of American Medical Colleges (AAMC). This does not include income lost as they pursue medical school rather than getting a job immediately out of undergraduate school.

According to Medscape's *Residents Salary & Debt Report 2015*, more than two-thirds of medical residents owe at least $50,000 in school debt, and only 20% are debt-free. It's no surprise that residents concede that not only is this a stress factor at the outset of their careers, but also that practice decisions are affected by the need to pay down this debt, as well as to make up as rapidly as possible income lost while preparing for the MD. This leads many freshly minted doctors to seek salaried employment with hospitals rather than go into private practice with its heavy financial commitment and greater degree of financial risk.

Cost Of Doing Business

Changes in delivery models, technological advances, payer policy as to reimbursement, and regulatory requirements have led to larger staffs in many independent practices even as physicians find themselves spending more time on administration than they'd like, which undercuts the time they can spend with patients, which is what generates income. When combined with the expenses faced by any small business, these factors have contributed to a dramatic rise in the cost of doing business.

Start-up is a particularly challenging time. It can take eight to ten months from decision to door opening, time in which the physician must make many subsequent decisions, all of them costing money. In addition to license fees and the costs of registration, setting up the business entity (PLC vs. LLC, for example), and trademarking a business name, the practice owner must acquire premises (usually rented), furnishings and equipment (office and medical), practice software (decision-support, EHR, coding, billing, compliance, record-keeping, and office programs), insurance (malpractice, workers' compensation, business liability, casualty, business overhead, and health insurance for self and staff), and staff (office and clinical — typically from 2.5 to 4.5 employees unless outside vendors are used for billing and other professional services). Income generation won't begin immediately, even if patients come, for the practice must register with Medicare and insurance companies before payments kick in. If the physician is not already established, there's also the time and expense necessary to attract patients through marketing or other activities. Up-front bank loans can help physicians with these start-up expenses, as well as give them enough of a cushion to make it through the period while income builds, but repayment of that loan, together with interest, becomes another business expense.

Ongoing, the physician must maintain enough of a cushion to handle financial shocks, such as changes in payer policies or networks, patient slow-down or abandonment, rent increases, equipment and software upgrades, rising cost of employee benefits, and increased charges for consultants needed for services the staff can't perform.

As even this brief summary suggests, the primary-care physician or specialist practicing in the traditionally independent manner has assumed a substantial financial risk at each stage of his or her career.

Career Path: Employee Vs. Independent Practitioner

Many physicians have very specific ideas of the appropriate way to practice medicine and have shaped their professional lives around this individual philosophy. The luxury of self-controlled practice, of course, requires either self-employment or working with other physicians of like mindset. That is an important reason for the fact that, according to the AMA study released in July 2015, 60.7% of physicians in 2014 worked in practices of ten or fewer physicians, and 56.8% worked in practices that were wholly physician-owned. According to The Physicians Foundation, more than 40% of physicians continue to practice in groups of fewer than five even in highly competitive urban markets.

The trend, however, is gradually shifting away from the traditional solo or small-practice model. The 2016 *Survey of America's Physicians: Physician Practice Patterns & Perspectives* (*2016 Survey*) administered by Merritt Hawkins for The Physicians Foundation had 17,163 physician respondents, of which:

◊   *20% practice in groups of 101 doctors or more (up from 12% in 2012)*

◊   *17% are in solo practice (down from 25% in 2012)*

Whichever group of physicians is surveyed, the general trend is consistent. Year by year, there have been decreases in the percentage of physicians who are practice owners and who are in solo practice. At the same time there have been increases in the percentage directly employed by a hospital or who work in practices that are at least partly owned by a hospital.

The reasons for this shift are easy to find. Private practice has become less attractive. Probably the principal reason is found in this disturbing statistic from a study by the AMA and Dartmouth-Hitchcock published in September 2016 in the *Annals of Internal Medicine*: only 27% of a physician's typical office day is spent with patients, while 49.2% is spent on electronic health records (EHRs) and clerical activities. Before and after the office day, physicians are spending an additional one to two hours on data entry.

That's one of the reasons why, much as physicians like independence, many don't like what's required to sustain it in today's environment. Some of those uncomfortable with the pressures of solo practice join group practices whose members share a like specialty or complementary specialties. This has led to growth in the popularity of group practices from the physician perspective. Clearly, it's more viable for a group practice to hire the highly specialized personnel necessary today for compliance, information technology, medical coding, coordination, and the like. It's easier, also, for group practices to justify investing in more-substantial premises, up-to-date equipment, and training. Also, group practices tend to have access to larger credit lines, a significant consideration given recent Medicare reimbursement-policy changes that have introduced even greater uncertainty as to both the amount and timing of income flow. To survive, it will be necessary for physician practices either to have access to substantial credit lines or to be so well capitalized that they are not dependent on full reimbursement within the usual time frame.

Becoming an employee ameliorates these issues, particularly greater financial risk. The entity buying the practice or hiring the physician, typically a hospital, is under many of the same industry pressures, but its financial position usually makes it better able to handle unpredictable income flow. Physicians who have gone to work for hospitals appear to feel relief in not having to sweat income flow and other challenges faced by the independent practitioner, although it's clear that the very process of making so basic a decision adds pressure in and of itself to an already stressful situation.

Whichever career path physicians decide to embrace – and the younger the physician, the more likely he or she is to go the employee route – the pressure to produce within narrowly defined parameters will continue.

The trend toward doctors choosing to become employees has repercussions across The Provider Universe. According to the *2016 Survey* administered by Merritt Hawkins for The Physicians Foundation, employed physicians see 19% fewer patients than practice owners.

Emerging Practice Models

In traditional private practice, patients made an appointment with the medical practice of their choice, saw the doctor, and paid the bill for that event (or had it paid for them by insurance or their employer). For years, medical practices found this simple, fee-for-service model worked well enough to cover overhead and provide physicians with an acceptable income.

Over time, as insurance reimbursements per episode shrank and Medicare imposed more-stringent billing requirements, this model became less attractive, and practices began to try alternative approaches. Some flirted with refusing to accept insurance and/or Medicare; some still do. According to the *2016 Survey,*

27% of the 17,263 physicians who responded don't see Medicare patients or limit the number they see and 36% of physicians don't see Medicaid patients or limit their number.

As payer requirements became more stringent, some physicians learned very quickly how to game the system by billing payers in ways that resulted in the same amount of income as before. Some modified their examination process to enable them to see many more patients during a day. Some abandoned "high-volume, crank-them-through, treadmill" approaches to care and turned to what is known as a micropractice or ideal micropractice (IMP), described by *Medical Economics* as "a low-volume, highly efficient solo practice that uses cutting-edge technology to keep overhead low and free up time for more doctor-patient interaction."

Other practices went in a different direction, replacing fee-for-service with the direct primary care (DPC) model, which does not take insurance and typically charges patients a monthly, quarterly, or annual fee to cover all or most services. A step beyond DPC is the concierge service in which patients pay a high annual retainer for enhanced access to the physician even as his or her practice continues to bill for specific products and services provided.

Some of these approaches work to maximize income and/or enable physicians to see more patients, others to create a more-satisfying work environment for physicians and more attention for patients. All present patients and doctors with tradeoffs.

Growing Importance Of Non-Clinical Support-Staff Specialties

Provider personnel can be divided into clinical and non-clinical staff. Clinical staff includes nurses (NPs, APRNs, RNs, APRNs, LPNs), physician assistants (PAs), radiology technicians, physical therapists, and others certified to provide medical services and whose functions are wholly or primarily medical. Non-clinical staff includes everyone else — all the people it takes to get patients in and out the door and handle general business functions. How large a staff is needed depends on the number of physicians in the practice, the nature of the practice, whether tests and treatment are provided on premises, and how many of the business functions are outsourced.

Once upon a time, even sizable medical practices had relatively minimal staff requirements. My first adult job, at the age of seventeen, several decades ago, was as receptionist in what was then one of the most-successful orthopedic practices in the Southeast. At the head of our little world were four doctors — three orthopedic surgeons and an oral surgeon. Supporting the doctors were nine people: RN, physical therapist, X-ray technician, three practical nurses, office manager, secretary, and — at the very bottom of that particular totem pole — me. The surgeons operated most mornings from six onward and then made hospital rounds, appearing in the office anywhere from nine to noon. On an average day around thirty to forty patients showed up for office visits (the practice didn't take appointments, meaning my real job was to keep patients from rioting as they waited, sometimes for hours). The surgeons made their own case notes in paper files. The office manager determined billing amounts according to a schedule unless told otherwise by the surgeons (who saw priests, ministers, nuns, medical professionals, and certain other favored patients for free). By today's standards, this was a barebones setup that generated significant amounts of income. If those physicians could have looked into the future to see the most-important non-clinical personnel required to run that kind of practice today, they'd be amazed.

The medical practice manager of today would probably correspond to the office manager in our setup, the secretary perhaps to the billing specialist, and the receptionist definitely to my job. In fact, of all the jobs in the office, probably mine would have changed the least save that now I'd be handling a lot more paperwork related strictly to sign-in and most of it would end up in digital form. Almost everything else would be new.

To begin with, for its volume and complexity, such a practice would need a Medical Compliance Officer, someone to handle every practice aspect touched by regulation. This would, according to PhysiciansPractice.com, include billing and reimbursement, HIPAA compliance, employment and training, Occupational Safety and Health Administration (OSHA) requirements, Clinical Laboratory Improvement Amendments of 1998 (CLIA) regulations, the Employee Retirement Income Security Act requirements, and "other healthcare regulatory areas, including Self-Referral/Stark Law and anti-kickback regulations." Even practice-website design is subject to regulatory review to ensure that it is ADA (Americans with Disabilities Act) compliant. Each practice has individual compliance requirements, depending on its nature and ongoing changes in the regulatory environment. Compliance officers need a wide range of continually updated knowledge covering most aspects of practice operation, how regulation affects them, the records that must be kept, and any reporting requirements that must be maintained. There are three ways to handle the need for this important office function: (1) hire an experienced specialist; (2) train a trusted employee; or (3) outsource it. None is cheap, and if the practice doesn't handle this correctly, the result could include fines, reduced income, lawsuits, bad publicity, and even suspension or closure.

Medical coding and billing (MB&C) are equally critical functions. The most common codes with which coders must be familiar are (1) the International Classification of Diseases (ICD), issued under the auspices of the World Health Organization (WHO), used to describe a patient's ailment, diagnosis, treatment, and outcome; (2) and Current Procedure Terminology (CPT), created by the AMA, describing the services the provider performed in connection with the patient's ailment. Between them, these codes serve as a common language to make it possible for providers to communicate to one another and to payers a specific account of what was wrong with the patient and what was done to affect it. Coding of charges according to ICD-9 was standard for years. As of October 1, 2015, all coding had to adhere to ICD-10, a more-specific classification than was previously possible. To maximize revenue, this is the general coding and billing procedure followed:

◊   *The doctor, nowadays using Computerized Provider Order Entry (CPOE), makes notes about patient symptoms, any tests ordered, diagnosis, treatment, and medication prescribed.*

◊   *Every support staffer in a medical office, hospital, or other health-care setting similarly makes a note of what he or she does with a patient.*

◊   *The coder translates these notes into codes that accurately reflect the patient's ailment, the diagnosis, and all services provided in connection with reaching that diagnosis and treating the patient.*

◊   *The coder then hands off these codes to whoever is responsible for billing — in some practices, the coder may handle billing as well.*

◊   *The person handling medical billing will then use the codes to bill the primary payer, most often an insurance plan or government agency, billing any co-pays, deductibles, and non-covered expenses to the patient or, if applicable, supplemental insurance plans. (Many offices require that patients pay the charges for which they are responsible at the time of the visit.)*

◊   *If the insurance plan, government agency, or supplemental insurer rejects any part of the bill, the billing specialist will work with the coder to address the issues and then re-bill, negotiating with the payer to reach an acceptable compromise if necessary.*

◊   *If the patient does not pay the charges for which he or she is responsible, the billing specialist will pursue collection according to office policy.*

Many medical providers handle all of this in-house. Others outsource some or all of the process. Whoever handles coding and billing, the process is more straightforward in theory than practice. There are, for example, over 68,000 codes in ICD-10, many of them very similar. Which of several similar codes is chosen can make a significant difference in the bill. With a serious procedure, such as cardiovascular surgery, using one code instead of another as to the precise nature of the condition can mean a difference of thousands of dollars. A good coder, while remaining honest, should be able to determine the code that will produce the most revenue for the provider. Coding encourages that as many individual acts as possible be performed in connection with patient care. Ever wonder why almost all appointments include weighing you and getting your blood pressure before you see the provider, even if you were there only the day before? Some of the reason is CYA or even super-caution to be sure you haven't changed so much in a few hours or days that prescription quantities could be affected. Some of it, however, relates to money. That few minutes with the measuring device and scale are additional codes capable of adding dollars to the bill.

Medical coding has become so important that an industry has arisen around not only basic training in how to code charges but also in how to interpret diagnoses and services so that they result in maximum revenue.

Qualified non-clinical personnel aren't cheap. The days when medical-office staffs were paid only somewhat better than routine office salaries are over. According to PayScale.com, here is average annual salary in 2017 for common clinical and non-clinical positions:

◊   *$90,268 - Physician Assistant (PA)*

◊   *$86,573 - Nurse Practitioner (NP)*

◊   *$72,038 - Practice Administrator*

◊   *$56,432 - Practice Manager*

◊   *$36,420 - Licensed Practical Nurse (LPN)*

◊   *$30,112 - Medical Assistant*

◊   *$28,163 - Medical Receptionist*

In addition to the money that must be expended to hire them, the highly specialized nature of many staffers means that the physician and nurse are no longer the only essential, highly trained professionals in the office.

Payment Issues

There are many things that physicians don't like about billing today, and they suspect that things aren't going to get better any time soon. Most disturbingly, the days of pure fee-for-service appear to be numbered, as is the practice of unbundling charges for billing.

In fee-for-service billing, the provider renders a service, bills for that service, and is paid, whatever the outcome. If the payer is an individual, then whatever the provider bills is the amount that is owed and must be paid or negotiated down. If the payer is Medicare or Medicaid, the provider is paid according to a schedule set forth that stipulates what will be paid for specific services. If the payer is a private insurance company or an employer self-insured for employee health care, the provider is paid according to a schedule that has been negotiated between the provider and the payer. In fee-for-service, each provider involved in a procedure submits one or more separate bills to payers. This is great for providers, as it enables billing methods that maximize the potential for profit. Payers, however, are resisting the continuance of pure pay-for-service. They prefer pay-for-performance. Pay-for-performance ties provider income to accountability, as it penalizes error, poor outcomes, and the like. In principle, this is a good thing, but its implementation will mean more physician recordkeeping, confusion as to how to measure certain aspects of performance, and potentially intrusive oversight of physician practices as well as of patient lifestyles. MACRA is refining pay-for-performance in a way that has many physicians nervous. (See *MACRA And Medicare Payment Reform*, below.)

Another hot payment topic has to do with the bundling/unbundling of billing. As described in *Growing Importance Of Non-Clinical Support-Staff Specialties*, above, physicians bill according to codes, each one of which relates to a service, procedure, product, etc., required for a patient's care. These codes tell the payer the patient's medical issue and what the physician claims was done to and for the patient. There are two ways that codes can be used for billing: bundled or unbundled. Bundled codes combine all the elements used for a patient episode. Unbundled codes list each element separately. An example of bundling would be that, when a patient visits the doctor, the practice office bills a single amount that is tied to a combined code that covers all aspects of interaction with the doctor and other staff, any tests, any treatment, and any products provided. Bundled codes are more efficient for payers, but unbundled codes make it easier for physicians attempting to maximize reimbursable expenses. For years, many physicians have used the unbundled approach to billing. With Medicare and Medicaid in the lead, however, payers are starting to pressure physicians to bundle billing.

Another form of bundling involves Accountable Care Organizations (ACOs) which, as a combined entity, bill payers for a set episode or period of patient care and then divide the resulting payment according to contractual arrangements between the ACO's participants. Sometimes it is the hospital that bills and then distributes the physician share, and sometimes the other way around.

Physicians are wary of both forms of bundling. Combination billing codes may not include a service or product necessary for a specific patient event and may not allow for the addition of a breakout code to cover what isn't included in the bundled code. This may lead to the physician electing not to provide that service or to miscode it to allow its incorporation in the combined code, both of which most physicians find unacceptable, in part because they appear to contradict the quest for improved quality and cost-effectiveness. Multi-provider or ACO bundling requires sophisticated contractual arrangements, careful monitoring, and the capacity to negotiate disputes, all of which involve physicians in time-consuming non-medical tasks or require that they retain expensive vendors or hire staff trained to handle such tasks.

Capitation is another payment model that holds risk for physicians. In this model, actuaries estimate the likely use of medical care for a payer's insured base and factor in the cost for providing the care plus a small profit. In the most-common model, the payer then pays the physician a set amount of money per month per member, whether or not the member uses the service. The physician then provides service to any members covered by the agreement without making any additional charge apart from those related to strictly negotiated exceptions.

This sounds like a good deal for physicians in that it is guaranteed income. The problem arises when the actuarial calculations are off and the total costs of treating the members using the service in a given month exceeds the total set payment the physician receives from the payer for all members, particularly when the capitation agreement has made the physician responsible for paying other providers.

Capitation agreements have proved tricky for physicians in the past, leading to financial ruin for some, which makes many physicians reluctant even to consider them. Once again, however, commercial payers such as health plans and large employers self-insured as to employee health care are in certain circumstances inviting physicians to enter into such agreements, and governmental payers appear to be reconsidering capitation as a way to contain costs. The AMA says such agreements can be made to work for physicians, but only if (1) the physician ensures that the terms of agreements reflect practice and population reality and (2) health insurers treat physicians as partners rather than as vendors to be exploited.

Another payment issue capable of disrupting income flow has been the Physician Quality Reporting System (PQRS), a Medicare program encouraging physicians and group practices to report information as to the quality of care given patients. The program was voluntary, but physicians and group practices who did not report satisfactory quality measures for *Medicare Part B Physician Fee Schedule* were subject to a negative payment adjustment. MACRA sunsets PQRS even as this is being written, and it's possible that practices already participating in PQRS may be able to use their experience as the basis for MACRA reporting.

Collecting patient payments is another problem. Respondents to the *Great American Physician Survey*, conducted each year by Physicians Practice, a division of IBM, report that 45.1% are having problems collecting large deductibles from patients, also that 23.5% are seeing claims denied due to a patient's non-payment of health-insurance premiums.

Cumulatively, the current environment is not one that inspires physicians with confidence as to future compensation. According to the *Annual Physician Practice Preference Survey for 2016* conducted by the Medicus Firm, the two greatest practice concerns were compensation and work-life balance. Physicians were most concerned with declining reimbursements, and this may be a contributory factor in the third greatest concern: work-related burnout and stress.

Ironically, according to Medscape's *2017 Physician Compensation Report*, in the six-year period between 2011 and 2017, "average income has risen from $206,000 in the 2011 report to $294,000 this year." Medscape attributes the increase to (1) higher salaries paid by hospitals to their physician employees and (2) improvements in efficiency and business practices by self-employed physicians. Looming over the reimbursement issue is the anticipated shortfall in the income of many physicians due to MACRA adjustments (see below).

MACRA & Medicare Payment Reform

The Medicare Access and CHIP Reauthorization Act of 2015 (MACRA) is bipartisan federal legislation that went into effect January 1, 2017, and has the potential to upend how providers deliver patient care by changing the way in which Medicare reimburses physicians, as well as physician assistants, nurse practitioners, clinical nurse specialists, and certified registered nurse anesthetists.

On the positive side from the physician perspective, MACRA repeals the detested Sustainable Growth Rate (SGR) Formula on which Medicare Part B had previously reimbursed physicians, a formula that attempted to contain Medicare spending by tying physician compensation rates to the growth in Gross Domestic Product (GDP). The formula was adjusted annually, and was on the verge of triggering a 21% reduction in physician fees when MACRA was passed in April 2015. Similarly, MACRA sunsets reporting requirements under several other CMS programs.

On the negative side, MACRA begins the Quality Payment Program, which requires wide-ranging data-collection, more detailed than previously required of physicians, and provides the strongest incentives yet for physicians to move from fee-for-service billing to pay-for-performance.

MACRA applies to (1) independent practitioners, whether solo or in a group practice, and (2) practitioners who aggregate and report their performance with others who form part of an ACO, PCMH, or other Alternative Payment Model (APM).

Participation in the Quality Payment Program is automatic for providers (1) who are already in an APM or (2) who bill Medicare more than $30,000 a year and provide care for more than 100 Medicare patients a year. For the Advanced APM path in 2017 the physician must receive 25% of revenue in Medicare payments or see 20% of his or her Medicare patients through an Advanced APM.

MACRA's Quality Payment Program offers physicians two tracks:

◊ *The Merit-Based Incentive Payment System (MIPS)*

◊ *Advanced Alternative Payment Models (APMs)*

Physicians who work for a hospital or are in another entity that qualifies as an APM can elect to report through either track.

Physicians who choose to report through the APM may earn a 5% incentive payment. Physicians who qualify for MIPS will earn a performance-based payment adjustment. MIPS participants must collect a range of measurements in four areas:

◊ *Quality of care and outcomes*

◊ *Use of health information technology (HIT)*

◊ *Costs*

◊ *Clinical practice improvement*

The 2017 information must be submitted to MIPS by March 31, 2018, in order for the physician to (1) avoid a negative 4% payment adjustment and (2) have the possibility of earning a positive payment adjustment under MIPS.

During 2018, Medicare will provide feedback to providers based on the information submitted. On January 1, 2019, 2017 participants who submitted their information by March 31, 2018, may earn a positive MIPS payment adjustment. Participants in a 2017 Advanced APM may earn the 5% incentive payment in 2019.

Participation in the Quality Payment Program is voluntary, but those who are not participants in an Advanced APM and who don't participate in MIPS, i.e., they send in no 2017 data by March 31, 2018, receive an automatic negative 4% payment adjustment. Participants who submit less than complete data for 2017 will avoid a downward payment adjustment. Participants who provide data for at least ninety days of 2017 may earn a neutral or positive payment adjustment. The size of any payment will depend on how much data the physician submits and the performance results relative to other practitioners.

In other words, MACRA will have a near-term impact on physician reimbursements, and that impact may be positive, negative, or neutral, depending on the information provided and the participation choice made by the physician.

In future years, physicians who stay in fee-for-service and participate in MIPS, will see a gradual increase in both bonuses for good performance and penalties for poor performance. Physicians who participate in a qualifying Advanced APM will receive a 5% bonus above Medicare payments and shared savings.

Whichever participation model the physician qualifies for, in the long term MACRA's Quality Payment Program will reward the best physicians and put the less than best on notice that they must improve — both of which should result in better care for patients and improved cost controls. In the short term, MACRA's recordkeeping requirements are especially intimidating, so intimidating that, according to Marc Mertz, MHA, FACMPE, vice president of GE Healthcare Camden Group, "For some independent physicians, MACRA may be the final straw that drives them to explore affiliation options." Other consultants agree that MACRA provides hospitals their best opportunity ever to recruit physician employees.

Apart from the formidable data-collection issue, the biggest problem providers have with the Quality Payment Program is that it makes revenue flow unpredictable, which is a huge issue for solo practitioners or those in small practices that may not be well enough capitalized to wait for part of their income.

The carrot for physicians being willing to be paid based on outcomes and cost effectiveness is that Medicare will provide higher bonus payments for quality care given Medicare patients. The stick is that the higher payments for the best providers will result in lower payments for the less proficient. CMS estimates that 87% of solo practitioners will see their payments decrease in 2019, the first year reimbursement rates will be affected. This should ultimately improve, but in the short term it will be a problem for many providers.

MACRA brings together in one framework payment policies, focus on quality, the management of patient care, cost efficiencies, and electronic health records. It is the most far-reaching advance ever in CMS's ongoing effort to keep Medicare sustainable and effective. When fully implemented, it has the potential to provide the most-basic restructuring of U.S. health care in decades.

For physicians, of course, its major impact is that it is the most-serious move thus far away from traditional fee-for service reimbursement and toward fee-for-performance.

2010 Patient Protection & Affordable Care Act (2010 ACA - Popular Nickname: Obamacare)

Stripped of its extraneous political baggage, the 2010 ACA is a combination of consumer protection, coverage coercion, coverage subsidy, cost control, and acceleration of innovation in health-care delivery.

On the protection front, the 2010 ACA returns greater control of health care to consumers through insurance reforms. As to coercion, the 2010 ACA allows for penalties to be imposed on most taxpayers who do not acquire health insurance. In terms of coverage-subsidy, the 2010 ACA provides for tax credits to small businesses that offer health insurance to employees and, for qualifying middle- and low-income families, a tax credit that pays in whole or in part for health-insurance premiums. In regard to cost control, the 2010 ACA: (1) institutes a pay-for-performance compensation model that will result in physicians providing higher-value care receiving higher payments than physicians who provide lower-value care and (2) establishes a national pilot program to encourage all those in the chain of providers for "an episode of care" to bill a flat joint rate rather than to bill piecemeal. Doing so entitles the group to receive a bonus from Medicare.

As to the acceleration of innovation in health-care delivery, the 2010 ACA

— as pointed out by The Commonwealth Fund — provides "a platform for testing new approaches to health care payment and delivery" in order "to improve value obtained for our health care dollars." It is this part of the 2010 ACA that has empowered the CMS Innovation Center to focus on initiatives such as Accountable Care Organizations (ACOs) and Patient-Centered Medical Homes (PCMHs), as well as to incentivize approximately 61,000 care-delivery experiments around the U.S.

The most-visible effect of the 2010 ACA's provisions from the provider perspective has been to make it possible for more consumers to get insurance coverage or to improve the coverage they have. This has pressured physicians who find themselves seeing disproportionate numbers of first-time patients with a wider range of health issues, playing "catch up" with health care they couldn't previously afford. Not only do these previously uninsured patients typically require more time per appointment, time for which payers are reluctant to offer full reimbursement, but they often resist or are unable to handle co-pays, deductibles, and out-of-pocket medical expenses. This has led to: (1) work overloads for providers even as all patients, 2010 ACA-covered or not, must wait longer to get an appointment and (2) declining physician revenues in relation to the amount of time spent providing patient care.

A less-visible effect of the 2010 ACA's provisions is the momentum it has put behind efforts to make providers act together to furnish comprehensive care for patients rather than viewing the patient piecemeal as part of an individual provider's business model. This is a trend that, while excellent in principle, strikes some physicians as something else undermining the way in which they want to practice medicine. Also, many physicians are suspicious of the pay-for-performance aspects of the 2010 ACA, seeing in them an attempt to reduce payment for services rendered.

The *2016 Survey* by Merritt Hawkins for the Physicians Foundation, reported that most physicians gave the 2010 ACA a "C" grade and only 3.2% gave it an "A." According to the *Annual Physician Practice Preference Survey for 2016* conducted by the Medicus Firm, 71% of the 2,413 providers gave the 2010 ACA a passing grade as compared to 83% in 2015 and 77% in 2014. Fewer than 3% of respondents gave the 2010 ACA an "A" grade.

Within the physician community, there is a wide range of opinions regarding the 2010 ACA. Its most-severe critics tend to be those who are older, politically conservative, better established, and in independent practice in affluent areas where patients tend to have private insurance. Those who view it as a generally worthwhile experiment, albeit with kinks that need to be corrected, tend to be younger, in the earlier stages of their careers, in practice in less-affluent areas where the 2010 ACA is critical for insurance coverage for many patients, employed by a hospital or other entity, and/or politically neutral or leaning toward liberal.

The biggest gripe that almost all doctors, whatever their political ideology, have about the 2010 ACA is the amount of bureaucracy involved. As one physician put it, "I became a doctor to treat patients, not to spend this much of my time justifying *how* I treat patients."

Incoming Republican officeholders vowed to get rid of the 2010 ACA, but thus far at least two concerted attempts have failed. Should a repeal ultimately succeed, some — or all — of the above may quickly become history. The uncertainty as to which parts will remain on the books adds to the frustration of physicians who've already taken on the burden of compliance.

The Elephant In The Room: Medicare

The importance of the role of Medicare in changing the health-care landscape cannot be overstated. In this summary of current forces affecting physicians the most, you'll notice that the carrot is often provided by Medicare, as is the stick. Through various initiatives, most recently MACRA, Medicare aims to reward physicians who improve individual care and outcomes for its patients, enhance a comprehensive care model, innovate to advance the practice of medicine, and manage to cut costs in relation to peers. On the other hand, Medicare will penalize physicians who underperform on quality-cost metrics in relation to peers. By its actions and example, Medicare is in effect acting as the primary innovator for the entire health-care industry.

Medicare has both the incentive and power to do this. As growing numbers of baby boomers become participants, advances in medicine ensure that they will use a wider range of medical services longer. The potential duration of those services and the fact that many of them have become disproportionately expensive in the last couple of decades became worrying, as did the amount of medical error and the failure to improve health outcomes. It was clear that something had to be done to promote greater quality and efficiency in the health-care system. Medicare has the power to do this through its role as the second most important health-care payer in the U.S., spending in 2015 a net of $546 billion, "net" meaning outgo less income from premiums and other offsetting receipts.

The need to keep Medicare financially viable has resulted in a full embrace of value-based purchasing. Tom Valik, in charge of CMS's Value-Based Purchasing Initiative, went on record more than ten years ago that the aim is the transformation of Medicare from a passive payer of claims to an active purchaser of value.

The combination of incentive and power is what has led to increasing pressure on provider performance by Medicare, the primary result of which is, as indicated earlier, the move away from pay-for-service toward pay-for-performance. Physicians may not like this, a fact reflected by the lobbying priorities of the AMA, but there is little they can do about the overall trend. As Stuart Guterman, vice president of The Commonwealth Fund, an independent health-policy research group puts it, "Medicare doesn't negotiate rates. It sets them."

The same might be said of how the rates are paid. Medicare increasingly sets billing and care standards. To begin with, these may be voluntary, as in pilot programs involving billing bundling, but as time passes those that prove successful will likely become requirements. The days of opting out of bundled payment initiatives, for example, are almost certainly numbered for physicians who want to avoid Medicare penalties.

Private insurance companies and other payers take cues from Medicare priorities and actions, so its influence goes far beyond its own turf.

Health-Insurance Company Consolidation

The ongoing consolidation in the health-insurance industry has led to a national landscape in which there are now only five major players, possibly about to become three if appeals courts ultimately allow two gigantic mergers to go forward.

The significance this has for physicians is that a reduced number of insurance companies limits policyholder choice so that the companies no longer must work so hard to appear to be an attractive option to policyholders. A smaller number of insurance companies can have several results, particularly: (1) higher premiums for policyholders wishing to access broad networks of providers; (2) competitive premiums only for policyholders willing to accept very high deductibles and co-pays; and (3) the so-called "narrow network" option that allows companies to justify cheaper premiums when they require policyholders to give up a greater degree of flexibility when choosing treatment providers.

Narrow networks can pose a major problem for physicians. Insurance companies assemble the networks based on several criteria, not the least important of which is provider willingness to accept a highly competitive rate for services and products. When a narrow network is created, those providers not willing to go along (or not given the opportunity) are eliminated from the network, and any policyholders who want to use their services pay out-of-network surcharges.

These narrow networks affect physicians in several ways:

◊ *They require or incentivize referrals within the narrow network.*

◊ *The tough fee negotiations lower physician profit margins for services provided.*

◊ *Being removed from an insurance company's network can almost immediately cost a physician a significant chunk of income.*

Whether the network is narrow or broad, dominant insurance companies have the power to hold physicians to stringent cost accountability.

Insurance-company consolidation is a thorny problem for physicians, especially since its outcome may in the end be decided by class action in the courts or by regulation rather than by physician-practice action.

Given the evidence cited in a study published in *Health Affairs* in 2017 that large providers have more clout with insurance companies, the growth in the power of insurance companies could induce more physicians to become hospital employees or to join forces in larger practices in order to have greater negotiating clout with insurance companies.

Complementary & Competitive Occupations

Once, only physicians (MDs) handled every aspect of patient care relating to diagnosis, treatment decisions, and medication prescribing. Today those tasks are shared with physician assistants (PAs) and nurse practitioners (NPs), who are specially qualified advanced-practice registered nurses (APRNs).

In the past, it was the MD who first interviewed the patient, noting symptoms, ordering tests, and the like. Some MDs continue to do this themselves, arguing that, in order to make a proper diagnosis, it is important to observe patients as they describe their symptoms. In many practices, however, the initial interview is now handled by a PA, NP, or APRN, who will take the patient history and order any tests that are indicated. Only then will the MD appear in person to make the final diagnosis. If the patient's issue requires surgery or further treatment, the MD will either perform the surgery and/or provide treatment or refer the patient to a surgeon or specialist. When patients return for monitoring, it will usually be the PA or APRN who sees them.

PAs have completed a fast-track version of the medical training given doctors and are licensed by the state to practice medicine in collaboration with a physician. Apart from acting as a primary in surgery, they are capable of performing most of the duties performed by physicians. Their exact duties in a given situation vary according to their workplace and the state in which it's located.

APRNs have at least a Master's Degree in Nursing and are certified by the state in which they practice. The majority of states require that they work under the supervision of a physician. Depending on their specialty, whether they have advanced to NP status, and/or the expectations of their employer, they may take health histories, order tests, diagnose and treat chronic and acute illness, prescribe medication, refer patients to specialists, and/or monitor ongoing progress.

The work of PAs and NPs and other APRNs enables MDs to maximize the value of their time, seeing many more patients in the course of a day than would otherwise be possible. This has the effect of both maximizing income potential and relieving the MD of routine tasks. Many MDs, however, are not comfortable with relinquishing what they view as core duties of the profession. "My PA is a lifesaver," one doctor told me. "But I miss the total patient experience. It's as if I've become more a manager of other medical professionals than a doctor."

There is also a suspicion among some physicians that the line drawn between full-fledged MDs and these "near-MDs" will become blurred. As physician shortages loom, it's likely that more states will allow NPs and PAs to perform most medical functions without MD supervision, effectively ending the long-time physician monopoly in basic medical care.

Increasing Competition

Every provider of health care, including physicians, is subject to competition.

Physicians compete over rankings and reviews, care outcomes, range of services offered, hours during which services are available, pricing, convenience of location and parking, customer satisfaction, and the effectiveness of their marketing and public-relations efforts in making sure that potential patients are aware of what they offer and favorably disposed towards using it.

Now, thanks to MACRA and other legislation and payer requirements, the competition for patients is being joined by the competition with other providers for reimbursement for services provided to those patients. The competition is based on costs in relation to quality, a worthwhile goal with which no professional would disagree, but the subjectivity inherent in measuring quality leaves many physicians wondering how fair the process will seem should they not turn out to rank well in comparison with their peers.

For independent physicians, this has resulted in soul searching as to why and how they want to practice medicine. Are they willing to join a group practice to make it possible to hire an administrator to deal with compliance and the IT consultants to provide the software support to meet ICD-10 and electronic health records requirements? How far are they willing to go to compete with the urgent-care center up the street that stays open 24/7 or the new practice whose web site is offering free initial visits? How comfortable are they with becoming part of the care chain required by PCMHs? Are they willing to go head-to-head with other providers on the basis of payer-mandated measurements, knowing that there's a possibility they may be paid less rather than more on the basis of outcomes? Should they respond to negative online reviews or ignore them? These are just some of the competition-related considerations facing solo or small group practices.

When The Practice Of Medicine Became A Trade

Competition has not always been a major concern for physicians, for health care was once thought above purely commercial considerations. For example, from the first Code of Ethics — issued in 1847 by the American Medical Association — until 1975 doctors were forbidden to advertise. Quacks might promote "wonder cures," taking out newspaper ads and parading through town in a top hat and tails, brandishing a signboard, but licensed doctors could do no more than appear on the membership rolls of professional associations or have a listing in the Yellow Pages. The Federal Trade Commission (FTC) changed everything in 1975 when it pursued anti-trust action against the AMA, accusing the medical community of "restraint of trade" for its refusal to advertise. This had a possibly intended side effect in that, according to the *Journal of Medical Ethics*, it "propelled the metamorphosis of the medical profession into a trade."

The aim of the FTC's action against the AMA appears to have been to turn doctors into "entrepreneurs within a free market," subject to the same kind of oversight as any other form of business. Ironically, with that 1975 anti-trust action, the FTC did little to control the quality or cost of health care but it definitely accelerated the emergence of the competition-driven, profit-maximization machine that the health-care industry has become.

It is interesting that the externally mandated regulations that made doctors businessmen, had almost immediate results in how the profession was regarded by the public. The Gallup Honesty and Ethics Poll of U.S. consumers ranks professions as to whether they are rated very high, high, average, low, or very low, and 1976 – the year following the 1975 FTC anti-trust suit – was the last year medical doctors topped the list.

Shortage Of Physicians

It's anticipated that the current shortage of physicians will accelerate and by 2025 there will be a shortfall of between 14,900 and 35,600 primary-care physicians and between 37,400 and 60,300 specialist physicians.

This shortage will be caused by these realities:

◊ *Many currently practicing physicians are close to or over a normal retirement age – one in three is over 60, one in eleven over 70.*

◊ *Not enough new physicians are graduating into the field to make up the vacuum left by projected retirements.*

◊ *There is a shortage of medical residencies, in spite of Health Resources & Services Administration (HRSA) programs like Teaching Health Center Graduate Medical Education (THCGME), Preventive Medicine Residency Program, Primary Care Medicine and Dentistry Career Development. As physicians must complete residencies in order to qualify, the number of residencies limits the number of physicians qualifying in any given year.*

◊ *Including medical school, internships, residencies, and fellowships, it takes years to train a physician who already has a B.A. or B.S. degree – seven is about the minimum number, so this is not a situation where an effort to qualify a large number of physicians fast is feasible, at least not physicians fully trained by today's standards.*

◊ *The number of patients needing physician care will create a need for approximately 33,000 additional physicians in the next ten years, over and above the number now in practice. The increase in patient numbers will come from population growth, medical advances that mean more patient conditions can be alleviated or managed, and the number of Baby Boomers entering the phase of their lives when they're most likely to need health care.*

The impact of shortages is already being felt. In the *2016 Survey,* latest in the series of surveys conducted biennially by Merritt Hawkins for The Physicians Foundation, 80% of the 17,263 physicians responding reported being overextended or at capacity, with no time to see additional patients.

The shortage, as indicated earlier, is being exacerbated by the 20-million-plus new patients that entered the health-care system as a result of the 2010 ACA.

Overextension leads to physician burnout, and a possible byproduct, also reported in the *2016 Survey*, is that 46.8% of the participating physicians plan to accelerate their retirement, which will further exacerbate the shortage.

Less Pressure & Greater Mobility – At A Price

As mentioned earlier, the traditional business path for physicians (MDs) wanting stability and a good income involved setting up their own practices or joining established practices as a partner. This allowed them to practice medicine in the way that they wanted; their patients were generally more satisfied with their care; and the financial rewards were significant. This continues to be the way in which many established U.S. physicians practice, but this is changing rapidly.

According to *The New York Times*, by 2014, "about 60% of family doctors and pediatricians, 50% of surgeons, and 25% of surgical subspecialties are employees rather than independent." There are various reasons for the willingness of MDs to become employees, but two of the most important, as already described, are relief from financial risk and disinclination to deal with increasing regulatory and administrative burdens. A third reason – greater mobility – offers even more advantages for the practitioner who becomes an employee.

Medical practice has not traditionally been particularly mobile. The independent private practice is geographically rooted. This has the advantage of a stable patient base in which patients not only return year after year, but also refer friends, family, and co-workers. Often, such practices own their premises or hold long-term leases in medical buildings. Many MDs find this satisfying and reassuring, others not so much especially given the rise of narrow networks that can destroy a geographically-focused patient base overnight. Also, there's the personal element. If the physician's personal circumstances change and she or he wants to move to a different geographic area and yet still continue to practice, the only option is to sell the current practice, which means giving up all the patients successfully served over the years even as the physician is attempting to set up practice in the new location. Also, selling the practice isn't always a simple matter and often involves the selling physician's staying around for a set period of time in order to integrate the buyers into the practice.

It's much easier for an employee-physician to move. When physicians become employees, they typically sign contracts for a set number of years. The contracts come with salaries, benefits, and the possibility to earn additional income through performance and other bonuses. The employee-physician typically has no financial risk and no responsibilities other than to practice medicine in collaboration with other employees, according to employer policies. Perhaps best of all, when the contract is up, the physician has the choice of (1) negotiating a renewal — possibly on even better terms, (2) signing a contract with a new employer located in a geographic area to which he or she would like to move, or (3) simply walking away. The only complicating factor is that physicians must be licensed to practice in any state to which they wish to move.

This puts a lot of pressure on still-independent physicians, many of whom don't want to give up the ability to practice medicine as they'd wish but are tempted by the opportunities that selling can offer.

"I didn't really want to sell my original practice," one doctor admitted, "but I wanted to move to an area with better weather and it was easy for me to get a contract with a really good practice. Moving was my first priority at that time. It didn't make any sense not to sell. Still, I think I'll regret it for the rest of my life."

Unending Advances In Medical Knowledge & New Technologies
The pace of medical advances and technological developments is continually accelerating. (See **Chapters Eight.** *Medical Advances, Medical Miracles* and **Thirteen.** *Major Challenge: Medical Advances And New Technology* to get a taste for what's here and what's coming.)

Ongoing education and/or retraining are required for physicians to keep up even generally with a medical knowledge base that has been doubling every five to eight years. Even younger physicians wanting to stay up to date will find it necessary to maintain a reasonably structured schedule of ongoing education. This represents not only a cost in itself but also income lost while the physician is studying, observing, or in class learning what's current as to diagnosis, treatment, devices, surgical techniques, and pharmaceuticals.

An interesting byproduct of advances will be the growing number of medical specialities made possible by expanding knowledge and new technologies.

Board Certification
An issue related to medical advances and the need for ongoing education is board certification. This refers to the taking of examinations conducted by specialist organizations that prove a physician is up to date on the knowledge required to practice effectively today in his or her specialty. Physicians can get a license

to practice without board certification, but the qualification — while not legally required — is considered the mark of a highly qualified practitioner.

Multiple boards administer the certification process, which varies from specialty to specialty. At one time, most of these boards required only one-time certification or occasional recertification. Now, however, they have "maintenance of certification" (MOC) recertification schedules to which doctors must adhere or lose their board standing.

Doctors say that the exam fees charged by many of these boards are exorbitantly high and the repeated tests difficult but irrelevant. In between the required exams, there are periodic questionnaires, which are also time consuming. Perhaps the most telling criticism of MOC requirements is that they ignore how medicine is increasingly practiced. Today's most-advanced physicians do not rely on their memory of abstruse minutiae to make diagnoses and determine treatment plans but access software-based decision-support tools to get the "latest and best" information on best practices. There are also medical apps like Figure 1 that allow doctors to share photographs and pool knowledge, as well as apps like Medscape, Iodine, Epocrates, and PubMed On Tap that bring together the latest information on medications and treatment.

A complicating factor in certification and recertification is the fact that many doctors are board-certified in more than one specialty, multiplying the frustrations involved in the process. The growing number of specialties made possible by advances in knowledge and the technology that supports them will probably lead to even more doctors seeking multiple certifications, each with its own initial and MOC requirements.

Practitioners particularly dislike that some boards work actively to persuade hospitals to blacklist physicians who don't get and keep board certification.

Recertification is such a hot topic that physicians vent about it regularly online, particularly on anonymous social-network sites like Sermo.com, where there's much talk about "meaningless" trivia regurgitation, over-the-top fees charged for exams, high failure rates on the exams, and the lack of any proof that recertification has any relation to better patient outcomes. Certification boards have begun to respond by simplifying some of their requirements.

From Mount Olympus To Competitive Fray

Physicians have always enjoyed a special position in the United States. That remains true today.

In March 2016, The Harris Poll released its ranking of the most-prestigious professions, and doctors topped the list, by far. Nine out of every ten American adults — 93% of those surveyed — consider it prestigious to be a physician and would encourage a child to pursue a career in medicine. Scientists came in a distant second at 83%. As for what makes the physician's occupation so highly regarded, The Harris Poll's Kathy Steinberg speculated in a communication to the Voice of America that it's because doctors — like other occupations in the poll's top ten — "are important to civilization and society in general." The Insider Monkey ranking of May 25, 2015, agreed, rating doctors #1 because of their power over life and death and "dedicating their craft and persistence to save and help people." The Gallup Poll released in December 2016 ranking Honesty/Ethics in Professions asked respondents to rate the honesty and ethical standard of different occupations as to very high, high, average, low, or very low. The top three rankings - that is, ranked very high or high - went to nurses at 84%, pharmacists at 67%, and medical doctors at 65%.

Such rankings are just one piece of evidence confirming that American doctors have always enjoyed, and continue to enjoy, enormous public confidence. In part, this is because of the depiction of the profession in entertainment, particularly on TV. There, by and large, doctors are heroes — smart, hard-working, dedicated to their profession, and devoted to the welfare of their patients. Even those shown as all too human or even cynical tend to have hearts of gold when it matters. Their image isn't hurt by the fact that, whether noble or sarcastic, brilliantly snarky or warmly friendly, TV doctors tend to be played by personally appealing, often attractive or sexy, and interesting actors. Think Hugh Laurie in *House*, George Clooney in *E.R.*, Denzel Washington in *St. Elsewhere*, or Jane Seymour in *Dr. Quinn: Medicine Woman*.

What gave such depictions their credibility was the fact that there was a sizable grain of truth at their core. Traditionally, there *were* doctors who were that determined to find the cure for a patient's condition, that kindly and compassionate, that much more focused on the greater good than on money or prestige, that innovative. There still are, but they're getting harder to find. I suspect that most doctors today would think my grandmother Maggie's internist of several decades ago a huge time-waster as he personally welcomed a frightened patient to his hospital, attended her cataract surgery himself even though it wasn't necessary, visited her every day to tell her all would be well, and personally called her after she returned home to see if everything was going O.K.

There are those who would say that the difference is that today's doctors are greedy, even cynical, attracted to the medical profession more because of the chance to make high incomes than because they feel a genuine calling. That's unlikely. It is simply too expensive and too much work to become a doctor, not to mention the fact that it takes too long. There are other occupations that bright men and women could pursue that would get them to bigger bucks in a shorter length of time.

The difference, it seems to me, is that back in the day it was easier to keep the ideals and priorities that led individuals to pursue medicine. For starters, physicians were part of a professional community that valued skill and intuition, had no need for self-promotion, and referred patients on the basis of their medical needs rather than the business model of their insurance companies. It didn't hurt that patients brought doctors their ills as if making an offering to a deity whose intelligence, training, and commitment they took as a given and whose diagnoses they usually accepted without question. It also didn't hurt that patients were generally loyal — once acquired they tended to return to the same practitioners for life. As for financial considerations, back then there was less suspicion regarding physician charges. Billing was a simpler process, and charges were much lower in relation to other expenses. This was because expenses were disproportionately lower — cheaper rent, lower staff salaries, more-modest decor, laughably small insurance premiums, fewer tests to give, basic X-rays instead of CT scans and MRIs, few government mandates with which to comply, no IT expenses, and less need for ongoing training to keep up with medical advances that arrived more gradually and were less disruptive. Back then, too, other medical professionals and even most patients gave doctors the benefit of the doubt when outcomes were not precisely what they should be. What it comes down to is that it hasn't been that long since the greater community still touched the collective forelock for its physicians.

As mentioned above, physicians continue to rate well when compared to other professions on polls measuring public respect or professional ethics, and individual physicians by and large are still admired and trusted by most of their patients. As a profession, however, the sad and sorry is that they've gone from the status of demigods to businesspeople subject to many of the same kind of controls, examinations, criticisms, competition, etc., as any other commercial enterprise. In fact, health care is among the most regulated of industries. And growing numbers of patients no longer view physicians as automatically superior beings

This was not the medicine many physicians signed up to practice; and, as their professional world has shifted around them, it seems as if they generally react in one of three ways:

◊   *Recognize the opportunity to be entrepreneurial and practice a more-innovative form of medicine that also offers the chance of making more money for the same amount of work if they can figure out a way to make it outside the current bureaucracy or, if still within it, to hit outstanding performance targets.*

◊   *Accept change with resignation and let themselves be swept along by whatever priorities are "squeaking loudest" at the moment — which may or may not be their patients.*

◊   *See "the end of the world as we know it" — themselves as beleaguered and unappreciated, with patients as part of the problem.*

In brief, many physicians are undergoing life-affecting stress. Some physicians and physicians-in-training react with the ultimate finality. The U.S. loses at least 400 doctors each year to suicide, doctors who over their professional lives collectively had the potential to provide care to one million Americans.

The Captains Of The Ship

All this matters to The Provider Universe and those it serves, for physicians remain the base and the core of health care in the United States. Payers regard them as the drivers of the machine and thus the most-important influencer of costs and quality. Other providers recognize them as the conduit through which patients are funneled to one or another course through the health-care system. As for those of us who are their patients, we trust them, and by and large they earn our trust. Physicians are the heroes of most patient stories, the captains of the ship that we expect to transport us back to health.

Chapter Nineteen.

Hospitals Having A Challenging Day

America's 5,600 hospitals are subject to many of the same pressures making the practice of medicine more difficult for physicians. The pressures affect all hospitals, including government, psychiatric, long-term care, and those classed by the American Hospital Association (AHA) as institutional, but are most serious for the 4,926 community hospitals open to the general public. These community hospitals in 2014 had:

◊ *786,874 staffed beds*

◊ *33,066,720 admissions*

◊ *$808,869,209,000 in expenses*

The different scale of hospital operations — more patients, more employees, more square feet of premises, more equipment, more of everything, lots more of everything — complicates hospital response to the pressures facing the entire provider universe. This is particularly true in relation to new technologies, where hospitals are expected to remain cutting edge without breaking the budget. Cumulatively, the challenges affecting hospitals not only have an adverse effect on the amount of overhead they carry, but also bring into question the sustainability of their traditional role.

Summary Of Challenges Facing Hospitals

Hospitals face very specific challenges in regard to:

◊ *Proper role of hospitals*

◊ *Expanding focus to population health management*

◊ *Physician-hospital relations*

◊ *Physician and nurse shortages*

◊ *Bundled payments — billing and dividing the spoils*

◊ *MACRA and Medicare's value-based payment goal*

◊   *Bad debt and debt write-offs*

◊   *Patient safety and quality*

◊   *Patient satisfaction*

◊   *Bullying — health care's dirty little secret*

◊   *Workplace violence*

◊   *Greater vertical integration*

◊   *Hospital consolidation*

◊   *Increasing competition*

◊   *Trends shifting away from what hospitals are set up for*

◊   *Environment capable of handling change*

◊   *From refuge for the sick and ill to commercial entity*

Cumulatively, hospital challenges relate not only to the amount of overhead they carry and medical advances requiring infrastructure reorganization but also bring into question the sustainability of their traditional role.

Proper Role of Hospitals

The evolution of the meaning of the very word suggests some of the issues making life difficult for hospitals today. According to the *Online Etymology Dictionary*, in the mid-thirteenth century the Old French word "hospital" meant "shelter for the needy." By the early fifteenth century, this was transformed into a "charitable institution to house and maintain the needy." By the mid-sixteenth century, it had become an "institution for sick or wounded people."

Modern hospitals find themselves enmeshed in the same crosscurrent of meanings and expectations. Long viewed as places of refuge for the ill or hurt, whatever their ability or inability to pay, able to afford this role because of multi-sourced subsidies in an era of lower costs, they have in the last couple of decades found themselves increasingly forced to assume a commercial mindset as costs have risen, subsidies have deteriorated, and payers have resisted reimbursement for the full cost of services. This has resulted in hospitals becoming more cautious about providing non-emergency services to all comers.

The Emergency Medical Treatment & Labor Act (EMTALA) of 1986 and Section 1867 of the Social Security Act ensure public access to emergency services regardless of ability to pay, but once the patient has received the immediately required attention, an ambiguous situation develops in which the hospital can transfer the patient. The question then becomes: who in the end is responsible for the indigent patient requiring further treatment but whose condition is stable?

The bottom line, of course, is money, with millions each year being written off by hospitals as uncompensated care. *Becker's Hospital Review* reported in September 2016 that, while the 2010 Patient Protection and Affordable Care Act (2010 ACA - Popular Nickname: Obamacare) has served to decrease the percentage of uncompensated care, the amount remains substantial — 3.1% of operating costs in the Medicaid expansion states, and 5.7% in non-expansion states.

Uncompensated care is written off by all sorts of hospitals, from safety-net Grady Health in Atlanta, GA, to prestigious Mayo Clinic in Rochester, MN, and Cleveland Clinic in Cleveland, OH . The amounts involved can be significant. In 2014, for example, Grady had bad debt and unpaid bills of $396 million.

Uncompensated care is a particular problem for safety-net hospitals like Grady — that is, public hospitals that provide health care to all, regardless of patient ability to pay. Safety-net hospitals find themselves in a vicious cycle propelled by politicians who appear to have little understanding as to the role of these institutions. To take just one example, a byproduct of the 2010 ACA was that it made insurance coverage more accessible and affordable for patients who once came to safety-net hospitals unable to pay but needing care. Before, these hospitals had treated such patients, collected whatever local or other subsidies helped offset the cost of their care, and wrote off the rest as a cost of doing business. Once the 2010 ACA kicked in, many of those patients now had insurance, which meant safety-net hospitals had a much-improved revenue flow. This new revenue meant the difference between survival and collapse for some institutions. At that point, other subsidies began to go away due to the increase in the number of insured patients these hospitals were seeing. As this was being written, politicians at the national level were attempting to repeal the 2010 ACA, thereby almost certainly ending insurance for most of those newly insured under its provisions. That effort appears to have stalled for the time being, but should it be revived, safety-net hospitals will be back to seeing these now-uninsured patients for free, this time without many of the local and other subsidies.

It isn't just safety-net hospitals that will be affected by repeal of the 2010 ACA. Many hospitals serving more-prosperous populations invested in providing the innovative care models prompted by some of the 2010 ACA's quality provisions. Repeal of the 2010 ACA would threaten the ongoing viability of care-delivery innovation without compensating institutions for money they've already spent in preparing themselves to deliver improved quality at lower cost, as required by some of the new care-delivery models. It would also add confusion to an already complicated situation in that it raises the question: how seriously should hospitals take government attempts to increase quality and reduce costs?

As this complex situation continues to morph and evolve, all hospitals, however different their situations or missions, face serious consequences unless they find a way to maintain financial viability in spite of revenue uncertainties. Evolving payer-reimbursement policies mean that additional revenue will probably have to come from nontraditional sources, which will prompt many hospitals to consider how they can leverage their existing resources in different ways in order to sustain their medical mission.

Expanding Focus To Population Health Management

Population Health Management (PHM) is essentially a public-private health hybrid involving the delivery of care to a group of individuals with similar healthcare needs. The similarity may relate not only to the specific health problem of the patient but also to age, sex, geographic location, employment, ethnicity, etc.

Rather than viewing each individual within a group as an isolated case, PHM takes into account not only individual-case specifics but also other determinants such as public-health interventions, genetics, social components (education, income, employment, culture, etc.), and environmental factors (air and water quality, housing, urban design, etc.). The rationale for this approach is statistical. According to HealthCatalyst.com, "80% of what affects health outcomes is associated with factors outside the traditional boundaries of healthcare delivery."

This approach requires the identification and aggregation of data from a wide range of information-technology resources to create a profile of a population that shares health issues and other characteristics. This aggregation allows an interdisciplinary team of clinicians, social workers, physical therapists, behavioral-health professionals, care coordinators, and business analysts to develop strategies for the most-efficient way to deliver high-quality care to a community of patients. This improvement results from incorporating insights gleaned from population analysis into individual treatment plans.

Theoretically, this broader perspective which takes logistical realities into account should have several positive results, such as:

◊   *Reduction in the frequency of individual health crises requiring emergency-room visits*

◊   *Maximization of the value of each service provided*

◊   *Increased use of lower-cost delivery options, such as mobile apps, online resources, and telemedicine*

◊   *Improving the overall health of the total population, leading to a reduction in the need for medical services,*

◊   *Higher levels of patient engagement, including self-management of health care and more participation in treatment-plan development*

◊   *Greater patient satisfaction*

Participating in PHM poses special challenges for hospitals. First, they know this means another round of major IT challenges, probably involving new software. Also, determining meaningful data at the point of care — rather than inputting masses of data with no context — is difficult. Also, physician buy-in can't be assumed, since physicians generally prefer to focus on sick patients rather than participate in long-term improvement initiatives. Also, specialists don't have obvious roles in the process. Perhaps most significantly for hospitals, especially when combined with initiatives such as the PCMH and community outreach, PHM potentially takes hospitals into delivery models and areas of activity for which there is no revenue-producing precedent. It makes sense for hospitals to take the lead in PHM, but how do you code it and who gets the bill?

Justifying the move toward PHM is the fact that some version is used in other industrialized nations that, when compared with the U.S., have better health outcomes at significantly less cost. American failure to use PHM seems to be the most-obvious difference in overall health-care results when compared to other industrialized nations.

Physician-Hospital Relations

Even when physicians are hospital employees, there are relationship challenges, for the independent mindset of physicians often makes it difficult to align their personal and professional goals with the cost-reduction and quality-improvement goals of the organization.

When it comes to physicians in private practice, hospitals face an even more complicated situation, for a long-established relationship model is undergoing significant and rapid change. Typically, in a world where most doctors were solo practitioners or in small practices, hospitals and physicians worked synergistically. Physicians saw patients in their offices and, if necessary, admitted them to a hospital where the physician had privileges. The cutoff point marking "necessary" was fairly clear — if surgery was required, if the patient was violently ill, if the patient had a condition about to get quickly worse, or if the patient was infectious. These were situations for which hospitalization was the obvious, sometimes the only, choice. Physicians billed payers for their services, whether inpatient or outpatient, and hospitals billed for theirs. As a rule, there was no competition between physicians and hospitals and little conflict.

In the evolving medical environment, where hospitals pursue vertical integration by employing large numbers of physicians directly and also by buying physician practices as well as other kinds of medical businesses sometimes owned or operated by physicians, there is a sense in the physician community that hospitals are setting themselves up in direct competition. This is happening at a time when physicians (1) are feeling greater competitive pressures and (2) have multiple options for patient care they are not set up to offer in their offices.

Insurance health plans have been quick to take advantage of the suspicion inherent in this situation by incentivizing physicians to utilize outpatient surgery centers, imaging companies, and other ambulatory services, using hospitals only as a care partner of last resource. This saves the payers money, lets physicians feel they're undermining an emerging competitor, and threatens a once-reliable hospital income stream.

This combination of competition and interdependency creates economic, moral, and legal ambiguities in the physician-hospital relationship. The uneasiness is compounded by the need for contracts related to bundling and Accountable Care Organizations (ACOs) and other emerging care-delivery models in which hospitals and independent physicians must work together. Marc Mertz, vice president of Los Angeles consulting firm GE Healthcare Camden Group, sees an opportunity for hospitals to improve physician relations by serving as a MACRA (Medicare Access and CHIP Reauthorization Act of 2015) information resource for practitioners on their medical staffs, perhaps even helping in the development of services to assist these practitioners with access to IT and other resources to help them get ready for MACRA. This kind of assistance might even benefit independent practitioners who admit patients to the hospital.

Physician & Nurse Shortages

The two occupations universally seen as most critical to safe and effective hospitals are physicians and nurses, and shortages in both occupations make this an ongoing issue.

How serious are the shortages?

◊ *As to physicians: The Association of American Medical Colleges (AAMC) in April 2016 projected that in the coming decade the U.S. will be short between 61,700 and 94,700 physicians. Those physician classes most likely to be affected by the shortage are primary care and general and vascular surgeons.*

◊ *As to nurses, in the United States Registered Nurse Workforce Report Card and Shortage Forecast published in the January 2012 issue of the American Journal of Medical Quality, researchers graded each U.S. state as to nursing shortages, reported that five got a "D" or "F" in 2009, and predicted that thirty would get a "D" or "F" in 2030. This rolling shortage is nothing new. In the last two to three decades, California, for example, has produced only 50% of the nurses it needed.*

Hospitals are addressing physician shortages within their facilities in various ways, including:

◊ *Buying medical practices*

◊ *Recruiting independent practitioners to become employees*

◊   *Utilizing limited-term contracts for certain physician specialties or for short-term needs*

◊   *Utilizing more physician assistants (PAs) and nurse practitioners (NPs) to perform certain medical functions once handled only by MDs*

◊   *Creating a more-positive work environment by: (1) having a strong physician leader to serve as a viable role model for the hospital's physicians; (2) facilitating a robust communications culture between leadership and physicians and among physicians; (3) encouraging hospital leadership to practice "management by walking around" that allows them to meet and get to know their physicians; (4) recognizing excellent performance informally and formally — thank-you notes and compliments go a long way; (5) coaching of low-performing physicians by physician leadership; and (6) removing a major source of stress by training physicians in risk management*

◊   *Focusing on long-term relationship building with independent practitioners who admit patients to the hospital*

Hospitals use a mix of strategies to deal with nurse shortages. Some focus on hiring from outside, others on growing staff capabilities by developing existing staff capabilities and using them in creative ways. All aim at retaining nurses, once hired. Some of the strategies being employed include:

◊   *Aggressive recruitment efforts: (1) regular recruitment events; (2) hiring of RN liaison who works with recruiters to ensure that a hospital is attractive to the applicant pool; (3) referral bonuses to existing employees; and (4) comprehensive compensation packages for new hires that include sign-on bonuses, tuition reimbursement, loan repayment programs, and the like. These work together to attract well-qualified staff, but must be consistently pursued.*

◊   *Short-term solutions: (1) salary increases; (2) limiting the number of hospital beds available for patients; and (3) use of temporary staff in the form of per-diem or travel nurses. These respond to immediate staffing needs, but are costly.*

◊   *Intermediate-term solutions: (1) development of existing staff through education and transition programs - nurses rotate through the medical-surgical environment and acute care, then progress to operating rooms or intensive-care units; (2) creation of dedicated resource staffing groups capable of immediate reassignment where needed; (3) payment of bonuses to employees becoming certified in a nursing specialty; (4) paying for nurses to attend work-related conferences; (5) creative salary structures that reward nurses for experience and demonstration of leadership; (6) assembling formal teams in which nurses collaborate to play an important role in advancing clinical quality and safety; (7) implementing seasonal workforce planning, which involves hiring nurses at high-demand times when admissions peak (holidays, flu season, etc.); and (8) achieving Magnet recognition from the American Nurses Credentialing Center (ANCC) — this allows nurses to recognize excellence in other nurses, and hospitals that achieve it have lower RN turnover rates and improved clinical outcomes, as well as improved patient satisfaction. While not immediate, these strategies work to bring greater satisfaction to the workplace within a generally predictable time frame.*

◊ *Long-term solutions: providing financial support for nursing education and creating a more-positive work environment. Nursing-education support includes: scholarships for nursing students at local schools, as well as co-op programs for junior and senior nursing students. Creation of a more-positive long-term work environment includes: (1) hiring more support staff so that nurses can function "at the top of their license;" (2) increased ongoing interaction between nurses and hospital leadership; (3) implementing "shared governance" so that nurses are involved in how care is delivered; and (4) enforcing improved hospital policies as to conditions of work that are a special concern to nurses (hours, bullying, workplace violence, etc.). These take more time to implement and may have limited impact in the short-term, but are more likely to diminish shortages in the long term.*

There is a school of thought claiming that there is no physician shortage, but only a failure to use existing resource correctly, particularly (1) telemedicine, (2) robotic surgery, and (3)NPs and PAs performing functions once the sole province of MDs. As to nursing shortages, various studies offer conflicting projections, with some claiming there will be no future shortage if real-world numbers are used for: those currently in nursing minus those reasonably expected to retire at different points plus additional nurses needed for anticipated demand. (A particularly incisive analysis of the ambiguities inherent in forecasting is found in Joanne Spetz, "Too Many, Too Few, or Just Right? Making Sense Of Conflicting RN Supply and Demand Forecasts," *Nursing Economic$*, May-June 2015.)

Whatever happens in the future, the current reality is that hospitals are already coping with both physician and nurse shortages, and the necessity is yet another issue to which hospital leadership must dedicate time and resource. Fortunately, many of the initiatives attempting to address shortages will almost certainly improve patient care because they'll result in adequate numbers of appropriately trained doctors and nurses who are motivated and experience greater job satisfaction.

Bundled Payments — Billing & Dividing the Spoils
Bundling of charges refers to the billing method wherein only a total charge is billed by a provider or a group of providers for a care episode or period of care. For years, hospitals and other providers have billed via a complicated item-by-item method, which tended to result in errors and duplicative charges that coincided with an explosion in health-care costs. The one bundled billing amount avoids such duplication, as well as doing away with any administrative or processing charge associated with each individual billing item. To the degree that hospitals benefited from such duplication and charges, revenue stream is affected.

There are two forms of "bundled" payments:

◊   *The first form of bundling covers episodes of care for a specific patient for a specific condition within a defined time frame. However many services or products are involved, the provider sends one bill covering everything.*

◊   *The second form of bundling — as in an Accountable Care Organization (ACO) — puts multiple providers together even though they may be paid under different methodologies. A hospital paid on diagnostic-related groups, for example, may be combined with fee-for-service physicians in a common financial risk pool.*

In practice, both forms of bundling may be incorporated. The goal of this payer-driven initiative is to encourage cost-effective care on the part of providers and to give payers a better handle on managing reimbursement. Instead of paying a dozen providers for multiple incidents of service in connection with a knee replacement, for example, the payer makes one payment to a single point of contact, which then allocates the money among participants. Typically, it is the hospital or primary-care physician who bills the payer and receives the payment and then distributes it among other entities involved in the care episode. Whichever entity receives the payment, the distribution is controlled by contract executed by members of the bundling group.

How exactly to manage both forms of bundling is a big issue among providers. For the time being, it's a learning process: what's included in a bundle; what triggers it; and when does it end? When multiple providers, especially disparate providers, are involved in a bundling group, what contractual provisions are necessary to cover group relations, especially as to reimbursement challenges and disputes? When a bundling group qualifies for payer bonuses by meeting certain metrics, how are they to be divided? When the bundling group is penalized for inadequate performance, how is the reimbursement shortfall to be apportioned?

Perhaps the major challenge is how to incentivize all providers in a bundling group to put equal thought and effort into how best to improve quality in their part of the process even while cutting costs. This is especially critical for hospitals with their large overheads because, with MACRA, Medicare has, in effect, "let the other shoe drop" by moving decisively away from fee-for-service as it ties physician reimbursement to alternative payment models (APMs) on a stated timeline.

MACRA & Medicare's Value-Based Payment Goal

In January 2015, the Department of Health and Human Services (DHHS) announced "measurable goals and a timeline to move the Medicare program, and the health-care system at large, toward paying providers based on the quality, rather than the quantity, of care they give patients."

In the old, traditional Medicare payment process, physicians are paid separately for each service whether needed or not and whatever the outcome. In this new goal-based environment, physicians — whether independent or employees — are paid according to outcomes and patient satisfaction.

Among the mechanisms in place to support these goals are Medicare's moving away from fee-for-service to alternative payment models (APMs) — such as ACOs, PCMHs, Bundled Payment Care Improvement (BPCI), etc. — thus encouraging hospitals and physicians to participate in these alternative models. Medicare incentivizes this change by tying increasingly substantial percentages of traditional physician reimbursement to value. The plan is that 30% of Medicare payments will be to APMs by the end of 2016 and 50% by the end of 2018.

Given that, according to HHS.gov, as recently as 2011 Medicare made almost no payments to providers through APMs and by 2015 made only 20%, this is an ambitious goal, and it's one that hospitals aren't meeting, at least for now. In June 2016, *Becker's Hospital CFO* reported that a Health Catalyst survey reveals that only 3% of health systems meet the target set by CMS and fewer than 25% of U.S. hospitals are likely to meet Medicare's 2018 goal.

According to *Becker's*, small hospitals with fewer than 200 beds are more likely not to be on track to meet the goal. The reason is simple: they have less access to capital sufficient to float them should they be penalized by Medicare for not meeting quality metrics in APMs, which are risk-based contracts.

For all hospitals, Medicare's structured move away from volume and toward value poses "between a rock and a hard place" challenges. If hospitals don't begin to transition to pay-for-performance within a continuum of care or bundled consortium, they may lose revenue simply by not making the transition. As they make this transition, however, and engage in risk-based contracts, they expose themselves to loss of revenue should the group as a whole fail to meet appropriate comparative metrics — and whether or not the group does this is, to some extent, out of the hospital's control.

MACRA accelerates the move toward value-based care for the physicians who work for hospitals, as well as for independent physicians.. In addition to replacing three Medicare reporting programs (Meaningful Use, the Physician Quality Reporting System, and the Value-Based Payment Modifier) and repealing the universally detested sustainable growth rate (SGR), MACRA ups the ante from the physician point of view. Through its Quality Payment Program, it offers physicians two tracks for participation via: (1) MIPS (Merit-Based Incentive Payment System); or (2) participation in a qualifying advanced APM. Failure to participate in one of these two tracks will mean penalties; participation eliminates the penalty and offers the opportunity to earn bonuses. Participation in MIPS requires significant recordkeeping and a stringent reporting schedule. Physicians who participate in an ACO or other qualifying advanced APM do not report data directly, but become part of the data reported by the APM, which provides another inducement for physicians to join forces with hospitals.

While the physicians most significantly affected (particularly by the record-keeping requirements) are those in independent practice, MACRA also applies to hospital-employed or -contracted physicians who must also qualify for one of the two Quality Payment Program tracks. Those who qualify for MIPS will probably be able to use their hospital's reporting measurements as the basis for their reporting. Those who qualify for the advanced-APM track must strive to meet group performance goals within the applicable APMs, but do not themselves report directly to Medicare. It will become more critical than ever for such physicians to align their professional goals and strategies with those of their institutions. What it comes down to is a lot of data and more than a small amount of risk for hospitals.

As the AHA put it in an issue brief of July 15, 2016:

> *Hospitals that employ physicians will defray some cost from implementation of and ongoing compliance with the new physician performance reporting requirements, as well as be at risk for any payment adjustments.*

MACRA implementation is a major concern for hospitals due to the approximately 250,000 physicians they employ and the 289,000 with whom they contract. As Ashley Thompson, Senior Vice President of Public Policy for the AHA, has stated, "You can't underestimate the cost of compliance with all of this... clinician eligibility will make MIPS and APMs a challenge specifically for hospitals to address. It also creates pressure for hospitals to participate in these risk-bearing arrangements." What complicates the issue, assuming the hospital invites employed or contracted physicians to participate in an APM, is the need to make a judgment as to whether a physician of outstanding quality will do better reporting according to MIPS, which allows the possibility of a higher bonus but also the risk of reduced compensation if metrics are not met.

Preparation for MACRA requirements as to advanced APMs will cost hospitals a lot of money. The AHA wants "an expanded definition of advanced APMs that recognizes the substantial investments that must be made [by hospitals] to launch and operate APM arrangements." Another area of concern for hospitals, especially those in problematic sociodemographic settings, is whether or not MACRA's currently allowable APMs incorporate what Thompson calls "appropriate risk adjustment" to allow for specific hospital circumstances. Much of this will be worked out in practice, but at the outset there appear to be many unanswered questions.

MACRA, which took effect January 1, 2017, puts hospitals yet again in the position of having to reassess their IT capabilities, particularly as to whether or not the hospital's information systems are capable of organizing and transmitting MACRA data according to CMS criteria by March 31, 2018. Hospitals that submit MACRA data for all of 2017 are eligible to receive a 5% incentive payment relating to physician services.

While MACRA presents challenges for hospitals, the complexity of the decisions it requires and their potential to affect physician income — a potential that grows each year — give hospitals an opportunity to strengthen hospital-physician relationships by assisting physicians not in an APM. One way this might be done is through the sharing of hospital-based measures; another would be in offering education to help clarify the issues involved in MACRA, possibly providing a guide to streamlining the MIPS reporting process. Also, MACRA offers hospitals both an incentive and a foundation to work more closely with employed physicians on performance measurement.

Bad Debt & Debt Write-Offs

There are two categories of unpaid hospital bills: (1) write-offs relating to financial assistance for those from whom the hospital did not anticipate payment; and (2) bad debts that arise from a hospital's inability to collect from other patients and/or their insurers monies owed for treatment, deductibles, and co-pays. Emergency-room charges are more likely to become bad debts because hospitals are required by law to provide urgent care whether or not the patient can pay. Charges related to other forms of hospital care can, however, also be a problem.

Uncompensated care is a major threat to hospital revenue streams. The AHA defines "uncompensated care" as "an overall measure of hospital care provided for which no payment was received from the patient or insurer." In its figures, the AHA includes both financial assistance and bad debts, but does not include other unfunded costs of care, for example, underpayment from Medicaid and Medicare.

A lot of money is involved. According to the AHA's Uncompensated Hospital Care Cost Fact Sheet of December 2016, "since 2000, hospitals of all types have provided more than $538 billion in uncompensated care to their patients." In 2015, the last year included in the study, 4,862 hospitals reported uncompensated care costs of $35.7 billion, representing 4.2% of total expenses.

As mentioned elsewhere, uncompensated care is a particular problem for safety-net hospitals, but affects all hospitals to some extent.

Patient Safety & Quality

Hospitals face special challenges in motivating physicians and other staffers, as well as in redesigning care processes and the work environment, to improve quality and safety. It's critical, however, that they address these issues in an appropriate manner, as all hospitals are required to report errors and patient outcomes as part of compliance with regulatory mandates.

Many hospitals also elect to participate in voluntary reporting to The Leapfrog Group, a national nonprofit organization founded in 2000 whose members include Fortune 100 companies, consumer-advocacy groups, and thirty-plus regional business coalitions focused on health. Called "Leapfrog" because its goal is for American hospitals to make big leaps forward in terms of quality and safety, Leapfrog has three initiatives:

> ◊   *The first Leapfrog initiative is its annual Hospital Survey, which collects and reports statistics tracking hospital performance — more than 1,800 hospitals voluntarily participate. It does not track every possible metric but focuses on those most vital to patient safety and payer value. It pays particular attention to the proper use of antibiotics, readmission, and Never Events, which are defined by the National Quality Forum (NQF) as errors in medical care that (1) are clearly identifiable, preventable, and serious in their consequences for patients and (2) indicate basic problems in a facility's safety and credibility.*

> ◊   *The second Leapfrog initiative is its Hospital Safety Score, which assigns letter grades to hospitals based on patient safety - more than 2,500 hospitals are evaluated.*

> ◊   *The third Leapfrog initiative is its Value-Based Purchasing Platform, which gives each hospital a "value score" based on data from the annual Hospital Survey. This score can then be used by health-care payers to identify and reward hospitals providing the highest-value care around the country by incorporating them in health-plan networks and/or referring patients to them.*

Hospitals report to Leapfrog as part of their attempt to retain market share because Leapfrog information is used by payers, like big employers and health-insurance plans, to guide their spending. The ultimate goal is for high-scoring hospitals to get more of their business and low-scoring hospitals less.

Leapfrog grades are also used by individual patients to find hospitals with a good record on patient safety. Patients are becoming more proactive in seeking out the best hospitals for three reasons: (1) thanks to the Internet, information is more readily available; (2) patients are increasingly concerned about medical errors and antibiotic-resistant bacteria; and (3) the rapid emergence of high-deductible insurance plans and elevated co-pays means patients are more likely to be paying a significant percentage of the bill themselves, which gives them a greater sense of ownership in the process.

In the short term, hospital participation in Leapfrog can seem counterproductive if the hospital gets a relatively poor rating. In the long-term, however, the aim is to use the Leapfrog metrics both as an indicator of what needs to improve in order to keep the hospital competitive and as a prominent means of indicating a hospital's commitment to ongoing improvement in safety and quality.

Patient Satisfaction

Related to quality and safety issues, but by no means confined to them, patient satisfaction has become more important due to (1) patient interaction on the Internet, (2) competition, and (3) customer-satisfaction surveys sent by providers or payers following hospital stays or procedures.

The Internet is an information-sharing behemoth that: (1) enables patients to leave reviews and ratings on a variety of sites; and (2) allows organizations and research groups who collect comparative hospital data to display it in a readily available format. Patient reviews and ratings online can be a wild card for many hospitals, as they are highly subjective, can be manipulated, and influence potential patients in their choice of a facility.

Probably the current gold standard for comparative patient-satisfaction information available online is the Hospital Consumer Assessment of Healthcare Providers and Systems (HCAHPS) Survey. The HCAHPS is the first attempt to standardize the nationwide collection of information relating to patient satisfaction. The survey's thirty-two questions include twenty-one patient perspectives on care. In addition, the survey allows patients to rate nine areas of service: communication with doctors; communication with nurses; responsiveness of hospital staff; pain management; communication about medicines; discharge information; cleanliness of the hospital environment; quietness of the hospital environment; and transition of care.

The HCAHPS was developed by CMS and AHRQ. The survey is sent by hospitals to patients within a few weeks of their discharge. Hospitals submit the resulting survey data to the HCAHPS data warehouse, where it's readied and analyzed by CMS. The resulting hospital-level results are reported on the Hospital Compare website four times a year.

There appears to be a sense in the hospital community that the survey does not necessarily represent the level of care provided to the patient but rather how well the facility *pleased* the patient, which may be two entirely different, perhaps conflicting, issues. The survey matters, because a hefty percentage — 25% in 2016 — of a hospital's performance used to calculate its Medicare incentive payment is based on the HCAHPS.

Bullying — Health Care's Dirty Little Secret

Bullying takes several forms in hospital-employee populations: shaming; humiliation; malicious rumors; condescending language; demeaning comments; insults due to ethnicity, religion, or appearance; throwing of objects; physical abuse and generally disrespectful behavior.

Although bullying is often manifested among nurses, a survey conducted by Safe Medication Practices suggests that doctors are most commonly the bullies. While some consider bullying as relatively minor and the ability to deal with it part of being an adult, hospitals cannot dismiss it so easily because it affects operations, particularly communication. Bullies are often impatient of questions or, when irritated, will simply hang up the phone or turn away. A bullying environment makes some people reluctant to answer questions or offer comments. Others respond by not returning calls. Others dodge confrontation with bullies by letting certain things slide — even issues related to patient safety — rather than speak up. In fact, a bullying environment is death to genuine cooperation or collaboration among team members.

Cumulatively, these behaviors affect patient care. It isn't just that those being bullied fear the risk of being assertive enough to point out problems or bring up opportunities in patient care, but also that bullies tend not to want them to and may actively discourage their saying anything. Also, bullied staffers are more likely to become disengaged and so may not be focused enough to avoid errors. Hospital management does not always realize the extent of a bullying problem because the nature of the issue means that employees are unlikely to report it. It is, nonetheless, the responsibility of hospitals to deal with bullying. According to *The Joint Commission Leadership Standard addressing disruptive and inappropriate behaviors/The CPI Workplace Bullying Seminar*, hospitals should:

    ◊   *Have a specific code of conduct in place that incorporates an explanation of bullying and associated penalties, and then enforce the stated consequences for unacceptable behavior — this includes documenting violations and appropriate corrections*

    ◊   *Regularly coach staff in how to communicate, with a focus on respect for others — this includes business etiquette and how to handle difficult people*

    ◊   *Create an environment where staffers feel comfortable reporting bullying, including establishing an official reporting procedure with direction to the person to whom staffers should speak regarding bullying*

Failure to deal appropriately with bullying costs hospitals money to the extent it increases turnover, lowers quality, or lessens cost-effectiveness. It can also open the hospital to liability if a staffer suffers mental-health issues attributable to, or made worse by, bullying unaddressed by the hospital. Bullying not only undermines efficiency, affects care quality, and erodes morale in the workplace, but also can lead to workplace violence.

Workplace Violence

Hospitals seem almost to have been designed to facilitate workplace violence. They employ large numbers of people, contract with many vendors, serve continually changing populations, have minimal security presence, and allow generally unrestricted public access.

This volatile combination of risk factors is exacerbated by other issues. Hospital patients and their visitors, for example, are often tired and under considerable stress. Hospital physical layouts can encourage a sense of privacy that makes perpetrators think they can get away with misbehavior, unobserved. Staffing may not be adequate for the multiple responsibilities involved in safe operations. Hospital employees are not always adequately trained in avoiding and handling incidents that might lead to violence.

According to the Occupational Safety and Health Administration (OSHA), U.S. health-care workers are four times more likely to be the targets of workplace violence than those in other industries. Data from the Bureau of Labor Statistics (BLS) indicates that attacks on health-care workers account for almost 70% of all nonfatal workplace assaults causing days away from work.

While workers in all parts of The Provider Universe are at risk, hospitals are the most likely venue where violence occurs. A 2014 *Journal of Emergency Nursing* survey from a large urban hospital system, for example, indicated that almost 80% of nurses reported being attacked on the job within the preceding year.

The violence may range from verbal abuse to spitting to physical attacks involving scratching, kicking, biting, strangling, even being tackled while walking down hospital corridors. And the violence doesn't end with minor attacks. Health-care workers are sometimes stalked, robbed, and even murdered. Patient attacks on hospital physicians can be as minor as a slap or as major as murder. Attacks may be spontaneous as when a patient is told something he or she doesn't like about treatment or length of stay and lashes out randomly, or premeditated as when the surviving son of a patient of a prominent heart surgeon enters the lobby, asks the Information Desk for the whereabouts in the hospital of the surgeon, and then locates the surgeon, pulls out a gun, and murders him on the spot. Sometimes the motive for workplace violence is profit, for example:

armed gangs have broken into hospital pharmacies to steal drugs.

Sometimes the source of workplace violence is a doctor — convicted serial killer Joseph Michael Swango, for example, is a licensed physician who has killed between thirty-five and sixty hospital patients by poisoning. Critical-care nurse Charles Cullen has admitted to killing between thirty and forty patients over a period of sixteen years in seven different hospitals by injecting them with lethal amounts of digoxin and poisoning bags of saline solution used for IVs. In both the Swango and Cullen cases, their employing hospitals suspected something was going on but did not report the issue to authorities capable of dealing with it. Nor did hospital references for the killers admit their suspicions; and these are but two instances of serious patient mistreatment that, while rare, occurs often enough to be a concern.

On a lesser scale of harm, there are nurses, aides, and therapists who deliberately cause patient distress. This kind of violence can be psychological or physical and may seem petty — the aide who repeatedly ignores patient requests for a change of bedding due to urinary accidents, the nurse who jerks out the IV with unnecessary force, the attendant who "accidentally" hits or drops the patient, and the like — but it affects many more patients than the more-dramatic forms of inappropriate behavior.

With increasing pressures on how much time physicians and other hospital personnel can spend with individual patients, it's likely that more patients will become hostile, making increased patient attacks on personnel even more likely. With growing personnel dissatisfaction, it's equally likely that more patients may be harmed by the action of disgruntled hospital employees and contractors, also more likely that there will be increases in employee-on-employee violence.

Recognition of the growing seriousness of the problem seems to be slow in coming, although some states are increasing penalties for attacks on health-care workers. Also, the CDC's National institute for Occupational Safety and Health (NIOSH) now awards grants for the development of prevention plans addressing the problem of workplace violence in health-care settings.

Greater Vertical Integration

Typically, hospitals have focused on inpatient care and the personnel and facilities needed to support that focus. Changing circumstances indicate the need to integrate services and care delivery throughout the health-care system, both before the patient enters the hospital and after the patient is discharged. This may mean contracting with other providers to align incentives or even buying other providers — such as physician practices, independent health clinics, rehabilitation centers, extended-care facilities, gyms, transport services, and the like.

Both owned and virtual vertical integration require up-front monetary and management commitments that can be difficult in the short term, and there is little long-term certainty as to how these investments will pay off for hospitals.

The impact on payers is often negative; for example, *Becker's Hospital Review* stated in 2014 that hospital ownership of physician practices leads to higher prices for patient care.

Hospital Consolidation

According to data from global consultancy Booz & Co., in the ten years between 1987 and 1997, hospital markets in metropolitan statistical areas with fewer than three million people became 27% more consolidated. The consolidation positioned hospitals to raise prices and spending. While the consolidation pace since then isn't quite as blisteringly fast overall, the trend continues.

Industry analyst Kit Kamholz, managing director of business consultancy Kaufman Hall, reports that in 2015 there were over 100 consolidations in hospitals and health systems, which is typical for the previous five years.

Why are there so many consolidations? According to Kamholz, the accelerating change to a value-based business model and population health management is making things much more complicated for independent hospitals. Also, cost management is a priority with probably every hospital in the country. It's critical for hospitals to align their operations around these new priorities and to do it as quickly and efficiently as possible. When independent hospitals realize they don't have the resources and expertise to do this, Kamholz says, they are more likely to consider partnerships. And the transactions are getting larger, involving revenue targets of $1 billion or more.

Realistically, consolidation between hospitals or hospital systems resolves one set of problems to cause another. In particular, merging multiple cultures and IT systems can prove difficult.

Consolidation may also involve hospital-physician combination. This kind of consolidation is particularly encouraged by the promotion of ACOs and bundled payments, the reasoning being if you must bill and be paid together, why not form one legal entity. Since such consolidations are often undertaken only to enhance the hospital's bargaining power, they are unlikely to lead to true integration.

In either form of consolidation, the impact on health care tends toward the negative. Consolidation between hospitals makes for a less-competitive marketplace. Studies show that, even though cost efficiencies may have been achieved, charges generally increase following consolidation of hospitals. Consolidations between physician practices and hospitals are usually not followed by quality improvements or reduced costs because that wasn't their goal.

Increasing Competition

Competition includes any type of facility that offers services once available only in hospitals. These include but are not necessarily limited to standalone facilities for imaging, outpatient surgery, urgent care, and rehabilitation. Physicians who would once have routinely admitted patients to hospitals for surgery now have other, lower-cost options, options that health plans and other payers encourage them to use. Physicians who view hospitals as competitors because of the large numbers of physicians they employ directly are often predisposed to use hospitals as the "facility of last resort." This means that a once-reliable revenue stream has been diminished.

Once, hospitals had little competition in the U.S., save among themselves. There weren't other alternatives for surgery or the treatment of life- or disability-threatening disease or injury. Now, competition comes from several directions, and may even be internal. Internal competition arises when marketplace pressures force the hospital to provide formerly inpatient services on an outpatient basis, which tends to result in lesser amounts of revenue being generated from services and facilities.

Hospitals have responded to external competition in several ways. In organizational terms, they may consolidate, set up their own ambulatory-care centers, or employ more physicians in the hospital. A very visible response is the move toward user-friendly premises and processes. Many hospitals are investing in attractive room decor and offering better food options and free WiFi. Patient rooms accommodate larger numbers of visitors. Friends and family members may remain longer hours, sometimes 24/7, depending on circumstances, and rooms are set up to accommodate visitors in relative comfort. Patient amenity kits include extras like eye masks and ear plugs. Hospital lobbies often resemble hotel lobbies or airport terminals and sport light, bright colors and original art intended to cheer. It sometimes appears as if lobbies are decorated by hospital PR firms, with rows of huge photographs of patients who've had great experiences at the facility.

Some hospitals are even set up to offer high-end hotel amenities — for example, uniformed valets and professional greeters, meals on demand 24/7, spa services, and chauffeured airport pickups. One justification for this level of patient service is stress reduction; medical researchers find this client-friendly approach can improve health outcomes. The main driver, however, may be the desire to market such differentials to patients (1) with the kind of health plans that let them choose where they go and (2) who have the money to pay out-of-pocket for services not covered by insurance. Another driver is the desire to attract medical tourists, who are footing their own bills and are picky as to what they'll get for their money. Hospitals with hotel-like amenities have higher patient-satisfaction ratings, a greater likelihood of patient recommendations to their friends, shorter stays, and lower readmission rates. They also tend to have healthier balance sheets.

A related development is the move by some larger hospitals to partner with luxury hotel chains to build nearby lodgings at which patients can stay prior to surgical procedures, during therapy, or for other hospital-related purposes.

A hospital service that many patients like is access to online portals that allow them to retrieve information about their ailments, tests, and treatments. They particularly appreciate the ability to schedule and change appointments online, as this is the kind of convenience they have come to expect from airline reservation portals and other enterprises in today's interconnected world. By conforming to general commercial norms, hospitals appear and are more up-to-date and businesslike.

Trends Shifting Away From What Hospitals Are Set Up For

General hospitals are set up to serve many functions. They have emergency departments to treat, well, emergencies — heart attacks, burns, accident-related injuries, any kind of condition that merits immediate attention. They have surgical units capable of handling surgical interventions ranging from the minor to major. They have intensive-care units for patients whose conditions require special treatment or continual monitoring. They have beds for patients requiring hospitalization but not needing intensive care. They may have outpatient departments that handle interventions not requiring hospitalization. Some contain rehabilitation units; others have floors or units dedicated to specific diseases or surgical procedures.

Their composition and organization reflect hospital history, present needs, and even their expectation of what will be required of them in the future.

To support all these functions, they have large staffs of both clinical and non-clinical personnel. It's estimated, for example, that a 250-bed hospital will have close to 2,000 employees. Because hospitals employ many professionals who must meet stringent educational and certification requirements, their staffs tend to be well paid. The BLS reports that in November 2016, the average hourly earnings of U.S. hospital employees were $31.31 (average hourly earnings for all private-enterprise employees in March 2017 were $26.14). Another major cost reality is that hospitals must spend large amounts of money on equipment, instruments, furniture, and fittings. An area of particular cost significance is that rapidly advancing technologies require accelerated replacement schedules on equipment, as well as ongoing training and retraining of personnel.

General hospitals are, in summary, all-purpose facilities for a wide range of patients requiring a wide range of services. As there is no way of predicting exactly which patients will show up needing which services, at least some of those capabilities are unused or underused at any given time. The expenses related to their existence, however, continue.

It's important to keep these cost factors in mind because, like any commercial enterprise, hospitals must be able to cover their expenses in one way or another. The cost to keep a wide range of functions operable is handled by incorporating overhead into all hospital charges. In other words, the patient occupying the standard hospital bed pays more to occupy that bed because it resides in a facility with a wide range of functions, most of which the patient may not need for a particular care episode. This means that general hospitals must charge more for specific services than would a smaller, more-specialized facility, and this at a time when value-conscious patients and payers have other options that offer similar or even identical services at lower costs.

Another factor relates to the less-than-outstanding record of hospitals in keeping their patients free from harm. In 2012, for example, *The Journal of the American Medical Association* reported that nearly 100,000 people die annually in U.S. hospitals from hospital errors, a figure much lower than that estimated by other sources but nonetheless alarming. Antibiotic-resistant infections contracted in hospitals are an area of particular concern. This means that hospitals have no claim on necessarily being the best or safest places to go for health care.

It is the combination of the cost/safety factors that is making hospitals the choice of last resort for many patients and payers. There are still times when a hospital is the only place you want to be. For everything else, however, there are alternatives. Why, for example, pay inpatient hospital charges for minor surgeries when they can be performed just as well on an outpatient basis for less money and with less risk of infection? Why go to the hospital E.R. (where it may take hours to be seen) when you can walk into a freestanding urgent-care center and get help faster and cheaper? Even if your insurance plan allows it, why stay in the hospital to recuperate from surgery when you can move to an intermediate-care facility that charges less and offers the exact services you need?

The bottom line is that patients and payers no longer expect one-stop shopping in a care facility, yet that is what hospitals are best at. Their ability to move patients across several levels of health care seamlessly is unparalleled. Unfortunately, payers feel they can no longer justify the cost of this versatility, and patients no longer seem to expect it – or even want to go through the bother of entering a complex system when there are simpler, faster, cheaper alternatives available for much of what hospitals do.

A related development is the fact that some of the new care-delivery models – particularly the PCMH – seem to anticipate that hospitals will move into the role of guardian of population health management, facilitator of the functions performed by others, and educators of patients. Yet these are not activities for which hospitals can charge, or at least not charge enough to compensate them for the loss of revenue from functions now being performed by other providers.

It's likely that this changing landscape lies behind hospital consolidations, likely also that some hospitals won't be able to figure out the transition period in time to survive. As for those hospitals that do survive, it' may be because of ancillary activities made possible by vertical integration or expansion away from strictly health-related activities.

Environment Capable Of Handling Change

As we've seen, health care is changing, and no one knows exactly what will happen next. This means that hospitals are implementing today's changes even as they try to create environments flexible and motivated enough to handle the changes coming tomorrow. The challenge, of course, is that no one knows which changes are coming.

The path toward change-friendly environments requires hospitals to strategize a structured approach.

◊ *To begin with, the hospital must identify the metrics to be focused on in terms of their importance - that is, the degree to which they affect the hospital's top priorities in relation to change.*

◊ *Then, the hospital must determine the best approach to align priorities across the personnel spectrum, from top management to physicians and nurses to Hygiene and Safety staff and even contracted vendors.*

◊ *Then, the hospital must conduct or otherwise provide ongoing training and retraining as and when needed to support those priorities.*

◊ *Then, the hospital must persuade all managers, employees, and vendors to identify their self-interest with that of the hospital so that they work to support hospital priorities.*

◊ *In particular, the hospital must maintain positive relationships with physicians who refer patients.*

◊ *At predetermined intervals, the hospital must measure performance in relation to the metrics on which it initially decided to focus.*

◊ *Finally, the hospital must generate regular communications designed to provide information within a consistent structure that in itself provides clues to the population as to how it is to handle the information. This communication must be designed to accommodate the different learning styles found in a large employee population.*

Cumulatively, all of the above prompts a relatively coherent chain of activity that should be readily accomplished by a well-run institution. Hospitals, however, are dealing with employees and vendors who may be already demoralized by the amount and pace of change. The typical hospital workforce is frustrated because its "normal" work flow is continually disrupted by changes in processes that result in short-term productivity losses even as the staff is being pushed to "do more with less." This means that any efforts toward increasing flexibility are likely to be viewed by employees as just another "flavor of the month." Also, communications initiatives are an expensive undertaking that can, if not handled correctly, lead only to a lot of money being spent to little effect.

Perhaps most alarmingly, attempts to create and maintain a flexible environment can result in the alienation of employees with other job opportunities at a time when shortages of qualified staff are already here or on the horizon.

It's difficult to predict the kind of changes that may be coming because circumstances evolve. As this book is going to press, for example, Brigham and Women's Hospital of Boston, one of the leading hospitals in the U.S., has announced that it is offering large-scale buyouts to employees (not including physicians and researchers). The voluntary offer is being made to 1,600 employees, or 9% of the hospital's workforce. According to *Boston Business Journal* and *The Boston Globe*, the buyout was prompted by the hospital's missing financial targets due to the decrease in numbers of surgeries performed, reimbursement challenges, and the debt burden from two recent projects - a $510 million building that opened in 2016 and a $335 million patient-health record system completed in 2015. It's significant that a teaching hospital as large and prestigious as Brigham and Women's – one of Boston's largest employers – is responding to immediate financial pressures by so major a cost-reduction initiative.

From Refuge For The Sick & Ill to Commercial Entity

We Americans have a special relationship with our hospitals. Most of us are born and die in hospitals, and in between it is to hospitals that we turn during serious medical emergencies. It is hospitals that we trust to repair body parts broken in accidents and to perform life-saving surgeries when disease strikes. It is in hospitals where most of our children are born and where we often share last words and handclasps with dying parents and grandparents. Hospitals are part of the fabric of our lives. Hospitals *matter*.

That special relationship has always been one of love-hate. Love because hospitals usually helped us, and hate because we associated them with pain, discomfort, death, dying, and probably the worst stress we can survive, especially when we're with a loved one going through an unexpected medical emergency.

Whatever we thought of hospitals, however, the main thing they represented to us was rescue and safety. Or at least this was true once upon a time. Nowadays, many Americans see hospitals primarily as profit centers out to extract as much money as possible from payers, be they private insurance companies, government agencies, or individual patients; and we suspect that they view us primarily as the mechanism whereby they can do this.

How we got from there to here is a tale of changes. Changes in who owns and runs hospitals, how they view their role, the services they expect to provide, the accelerating pace of medical advances, how they're paid and by whom, the competitive and regulatory environment in which they function, the expectations of the public they serve, the staffing and infrastructure required to underpin this evolving role, and the degree to which they are valued and subsidized by the community in which they're located.

The Ocean Liners Of Health Care

Once, hospitals viewed their work as a mission to serve; now necessity has made them business enterprises buried in IT minutiae, their operations pulled this way and that by legislation, regulation, increasing costs, payer resistance, and political ambiguity. Any inability, as business enterprises, to prioritize creating an environment that can handle change may turn them into the victims of the ongoing health-care revolution. It's easier to turn a rowboat than an ocean liner, and hospitals are the liners of health care.

Of course, sometimes you need a liner — anyone willing to head for the furthest reaches of a stormy ocean in a canoe? Anyone know of anywhere other than a hospital where all the resources exist that are needed to diagnose a complex medical issue, create a treatment plan, implement the plan, monitor the result, and deal with anything unexpected that happens along the way? Anyone willing to trust their health to a system that doesn't include strong hospitals?

Chapter Twenty.

Nurses In An Identity Crisis

Nurses are the face of the U.S. provider universe, the members of its workforce with whom patients and their families most frequently interact. Nurses are well respected by the population at large — the Gallup poll released December 2016 ranking Honesty/Ethics in Professions rates them #1, with 84% of respondents rating them as Very High/High. Numerically, they are by far the largest segment of the health-care workforce in the U.S. There are many kinds of nurses: staff nurses, also known as LPNs; registered nurses (RNs); advanced-practice nurses (APRNs); nurse practitioners (NPs); administrative nurses; and educator nurses, to name some of the most common.

Nurses work not just on hospital floors and in physician practices but in many settings: operating rooms; delivery rooms; intensive-care units; hospices; ships; helicopters; planes; ambulatory-care centers; nursing homes; emergency rooms; courtrooms; the armed forces; psychiatric centers; geriatric centers; community centers; prisons; schools; laboratories and research centers; and in every place patients may need care or employers require their nursing-related services, as well as in college classrooms training other nurses.

Most health-care practitioners work in all or many of these places, but the difference with nurses in clinical settings is that others tend to perform a specific task and leave, while nurses remain to give ongoing care. It is nurses who check on patients and their families — many times an hour in critical care. They run tests, record symptoms, assess ailments, administer medications and treatments, change IVs, answer questions, and offer information about ongoing treatment. They provide psychological support and add to the patient's physical comfort. It is nurses who keep things going in health care.

Nurses form the core of The Provider Universe, giving it not only its impetus but also much of its personality and heart; and nursing is a profession that offers much to those who enter it.

Registered nurses form the single largest segment of health care. According to the *Occupational Outlook Handbook (OOH)*, in 2014 - there were 2,751,000 RNs, with median annual pay of $66,640. The *OOH* anticipates job growth of 16% between 2014 and 2024, which is much faster than average for all job fields. This anticipated increase will add another 439,300 individuals to RN employment.

RNs can, if they choose and acquire the appropriate training and/or experience, pursue various specialties, for example: addiction; cardiovascular; critical care; genetics; neonatology; nephrology; rehabilitation; and advanced practice. There are strong professional associations, in particular the American Nurses Association (ANA) and the National Student Nurses Association (NSNA), that perform research into areas of concern, disseminate information about the state of the profession, and represent the interests of nursing in the broader community,

Nursing offers individuals with suitable abilities and temperaments the chance to exercise all of their attributes and skills – intelligence, education, training, energy, curiosity, empathy, and management abilities. Nursing is, moreover, a job that offers incredible mobility. A properly credentialed nurse can find work just about anywhere in the U.S. and abroad.

In spite of opportunity, mobility, and challenge, however, many members of the nursing profession are frustrated with their lot. In what amounts to more or less a generation of change, nurses have seen the focus of their profession shift from patients to processes, the nature of their relationships with co-workers – particularly doctors – become increasingly ambiguous, and the demands of their professional duties expand far out of proportion to the financial reward and recognition they receive.

Summary Of Issues Relating To Nurses In An Identity Crisis

Many issues play a role in what is going on in American nursing in 2017, among them:

♢   *Evolution of traditional role*

♢   *Ambiguity in physician-nurse roles and relationships*

♢   *Nurse Practitioners vs. MDs*

♢   *Hours and pay*

♢   *Shortage of nursing staff*

♢   *Exposure to diseases and hazardous chemicals*

♢   *Patient liaison difficulties*

♢   *Workplace violence*

♢   *Lack of adequate policies for guidance in the handling of real-world issues*

♢   *Miscommunication with patients due to language difficulties*

♢   *Lack of respect in relation to responsibilities*

◊   *Expansion of nursing skill sets*

◊   *The emerging nurse persona*

All of the above are changing the nature of nursing today.

Evolution Of Traditional Role

Long viewed by many in the health-care industry as the handmaidens of physicians, their success judged by the efficiency with which they followed orders, nurses find that much more is expected of them today. Moreover, they are themselves increasingly disinclined to remain within the occupation's traditional confines.

Even as doctors in private practice assume duties that incorporate elements of both business and medicine and hospitals are confronted by multiple challenges to their traditional role, it is nurses who bear much of the brunt of change.

Traditionally, nurses spent most of their time serving immediate patient needs. The growing complexity of the hospital and medical-office environment now requires that they spend increasing amounts of time on paperwork and other tasks not directly related to patient care. A 2014 article in *The Wall Street Journal* estimated that, in a twelve-hour shift, nurses may spend as little as two hours on patient care. In the portion of their day dedicated to care, they are tasked with managing and performing processes at least as much as interacting with patients.

The one-time "handmaidens of physicians" must now align their knowledge, skills, and attitudes with what's required in their practice environments. They must be able to work effectively with other professionals in multiple health-care settings. In addition to their traditional role as care provider they must now be able to handle case and practice leadership and case management. They must stay abreast of advanced technologies affecting patient care. They must understand the nuances of alternate care-delivery models and their role in making them work. On top of that, they're often expected to provide health and disease-prevention information to patients. That's a lot of responsibility, requiring a wide range of skill sets. In many ways, nurses welcome this; in others, they have reservations.

As one long-time nurse at a large, Midwestern hospital puts it, "When I started, we more or less took orders. That left a lot to be desired. Taking orders was very limited. I like the idea of being able to use more of my abilities and new technologies to help patients through difficult times. I even like the idea of helping the hospital improve its standing. What I don't like is that I get no additional respect and little, if any, additional money for these increased responsibilities. It's as if we're where the buck stops and starts to shrink. I'm tired of being taken for granted. When things go right, the doctors and administrators take the credit. When they go wrong, we're the ones they blame, and everything gets upended again."

Clearly, the nursing world has transformed, yet attitudes toward nurses and compensation have not followed this shift.

Ambiguity In Changing Physician-Nurse Roles & Relationships

Traditionally, physicians and nurses played clearly defined roles in health care.

Physicians diagnosed and performed surgery; nurses provided aid and physical treatment. Their fields of operations differed as well in that doctors worked within their specialty while nurses could work across several wards or units, limited only by their job description in a specific hospital.

Their attitudes toward their patients tended to differ. Physicians performed best when they maintained a certain emotional distance, focusing on patient ailments rather than patient as person because of the need to remain analytical. Nurses, on the other hand, often enjoyed a closer personal relationship with patients because of the amount of direct contact they had, contact that involved specific duties in relation to patient needs already determined by the physician.

As they continued in their careers, physicians were expected not only to benefit from experience but to remain academically up to date as well, while nurses tended to rely more on experience and less on formal retraining.

Perhaps the greatest difference in their job functions, however, had to do with the assumption of ultimate responsibility for medical outcomes. Here, the physician was the one who made the decisions and issued the orders, while the nurse followed his instructions. It was this difference — and, probably, the fact that traditionally most physicians were male and most nurses female — that has accounted for the large difference in the amount of money physicians and nurses earn and in the respect accorded each profession.

That world in which physicians automatically led and nurses more or less automatically followed is, however, changing. Today, nurses get more training than before, both at the outset and throughout their careers, and expect to use it. Also, hospitals expect nurses to follow physicians' orders within the context of the institution's rules and priorities. All of this creates an overlap of authority.

Studies suggest that the two biggest problems between physicians and nurses have to do with communication and understanding. The communication issue develops because, even when supposedly working in teams, physicians don't routinely involve nurses in rounds or inform them when patient objectives are altered. Perhaps even more worrying is that many physicians appear to finish their medical training without having acquired the ability to see situations from the nurse's perspective. Physicians sometimes even hold mistaken notions as to the role of the nurse in the contemporary medical scene. This sets up unreasonable expectations and may even lead to confusion. What's needed are two things: (1) an environment of mutual trust in which both physicians and nurses can share information and question one another without suspicion or animosity; and (2) a better understanding on the part of physicians as to the training required to become a nurse and what that training makes nurses capable of doing in today's more-sophisticated and demanding provider universe.

It is a particular grievance in the nursing community that they not only continue to be paid significantly less than physicians but also their contribution is not adequately recognized by physicians, employers, the community, and even the patients they serve. Patients may like nurses better, but on a day-to-day basis, it is the appearance of the physician that makes most of them pay attention and do as they're told.

Ideally, physicians and nurses work as part of a team with other medical professionals to provide the best outcome for patients. Each member of the team should have a right to make suggestions that influence patient care. While productive in terms of patient outcomes, this is not a situation with which many physicians are comfortable, especially physicians trained in a different tradition, and nurses sometimes find themselves working alongside physicians who resent their changing role.

Nurse Practitioners & APRNs Vs. MDs

Uncomfortable as they may be with assertive RNs and LPNs, many physicians save their greatest reservations for nurse practitioners (NPs) and other APRNs. In fact, one physician told me that a few years ago he set off what amounted to a medical food fight in a seminar by suggesting that MDs would benefit from focusing less on trying to limit the role of NPs and other APRNs and more on figuring out how to use their skills to make life easier and more productive for physicians.

APRNs have obtained at least a Master's degree in Nursing. NPs are APRNs who have at least a Master of Science in Nursing — a PhD or DNP (Doctor of Nursing Practice) will soon be required — and up to 700 additional hours of supervised clinical work to qualify them to manage acute and chronic medical conditions. They must recertify with the American Association of Nurse Practitioners (AANP) or another certification entity every five years. Recertification requires at least 1,000 hours of clinical practice in the preceding five years and seventy-five hours of continuing education relevant to the NP's role and specialty.

In professional terms, NPs can take histories, give medical exams, and order diagnostic tests. They can, moreover, diagnose medical problems and order treatments. They can prescribe medication. Many NPs are the patient's primary provider. Given the appropriate training and experience, NPs can even specialize.

This puts them in territory once occupied solely by MDs, especially in those fifteen-plus states that do not require their primary-care activities to be supervised by a physician. (Most states require that NPs work with a physician under a written practice agreement, but this is likely to change.)

New opportunities for NPs and APRNs are already here and will probably continue to grow. They have been recognized as a provider of primary-care services with the potential to lead within the new care-delivery models. Nurse-Managed Health Clinics (NMHCs), for example, are nurse-practice setups led by NPs or other APRNs affiliated with an approved institution. They serve vulnerable populations by providing comprehensive primary care and wellness services in a cost-effective manner appealing to payers. A limitation to the effectiveness of APRNs is the failure of some hospitals and other employers to provide the circumstances that allow them to practice to the level of their qualifications.

There is expert validation for the use of NPs. In 2000, the Institute of Medicine (IOM) recommended that NPs should be allowed to practice "to the full extent of their education and training," leading medical teams and practices and being paid at the same rate as physicians for the same work. The IOM's stamp of approval for NPs is significant, but other medical-industry organizations have reservations. The American Medical Association (AMA), for example, which represents the interests of physicians, disagrees. The AMA and its membership say there isn't enough data to justify allowing NPs this degree of latitude. Most doctors claim that only they, with their more-intensive training and long-honed intuition, are capable of providing an adequate level of care and that, in fact, utilizing NPs instead of MDs can actually harm patients.

It's likely that physicians are waging an unwinnable war against NPs and other APRNs, because just about everyone else already supports the expansion of their functions. Payers like NPs because lower payments traditionally associated with the care they provide help with cost controls. Geographic areas without adequate numbers of physicians like NPs because they provide medical care that would otherwise be unavailable. Facilities that provide walk-in care for minor injuries and ailments like NPs because they provide an economical alternative to the employment of physicians. Nurses themselves like the possibility of becoming NPs because it gives them an alternative career path and added scope for their intelligence, abilities, and dedication.

According to the BLS, in 2014 there were 126,900 NPs. When added to 38,200 nurse anesthetists and 5,300 nurse midwives practicing in that year, this means that 170,400 jobs once held by MDs became the purview of APRNs. Their combined number is expected to rise to 223,800 by 2024, and this 31% increase makes many physicians think that society will continue to seek what MDs view as less-qualified alternatives simply to save money.

This rise of APRNs has had a certain amount of impact on nurse interactions with others in their work environment. Even those nurses who do not elect or do not have the opportunity to become APRNs are aware that the possibility exists, and this inevitably affects attitudes. While nurses continue to support the physician role, they now expect more input and that more attention be paid to their expertise.

Hours & Pay

Hours and shift schedules are a particular source of contention in nursing. Working hours are long and shifts may be badly timed, often back to back. Both factors contribute to fatigue, stress, and uncertainty. One solution is that hospitals allow nurses a say in how work is organized and assigned. If the hours-shift issue is not resolved, it can lead to burnout, which undermines care quality and safety and which may also lead some nurses to quit.

Nurse pay varies significantly, depending on specialty, employer, experience level, and geographical location. According to PayScale.com, a RN earns an average wage of $28.15 per hour or $1,126.00 for a forty-hour week, but this can vary from $21.79-$39.85 per hour plus, in some instances, bonuses, commissions, profit sharing, hourly tips, and overtime. The *Occupational Outlook Handbook* cites a somewhat higher median pay of $66,640 per year.

That doesn't sound bad, but nurses feel that compensation is low in relation to responsibilities and in comparison with others in the health-care industry. Compare the $58,552 average annual base salary for RNs cited by PayScale.com to the $167,321 cited by the same source for family physicians. Nurses don't question that doctors should be paid in relation to their training, skills, and experience; what they do question is why nurses aren't paid more in relation to theirs. An especially irritating trend is for physician assistants (PAs), who are usually male, to be paid more than NPs.

Pay for NPs is a particularly contentious issue. Since their preference for NPs for the treatment of simple conditions is based on lower pay scales, payers resist increases in NP compensation. Also, most doctors strenuously oppose NPs being paid salaries comparable to those they receive, even for comparable duties with comparable outcomes. To this, NPs can legitimately respond that it is only fair that for additional responsibilities they receive corresponding increases in pay.

Shortage Of Nursing Staff

As remarked earlier, nurses — who remain overwhelmingly female — are the largest segment of the U.S. health-care workforce, and nursing is one of the fastest-growing occupations in the country. In spite of these numbers, demand for nurses is greater than supply.

The shortage of nurses is decades in the making, but it's worsened in the past few years, the most obvious reasons being the increase in chronic disease and the fact that an aging American population with high expectations as to medical treatment is placing ever-growing demands on the system. Other reasons for demand exceeding supply include:

◊ *Women seeking professional careers have other choices that may pay better and require less training, and not enough men have entered nursing to compensate.*

◊ *Nursing is no longer as attractive an occupation as it once was due to long hours, stressful working conditions, inadequate pay scales in relation to current responsibilities, and lack of respect. This leads to burnout, which prompts some nurses to leave the occupation.*

◊   *Nurses are reaching retirement age at an accelerating pace. One-third of the current nursing workforce will be old enough to retire in the next ten to fifteen years.*

◊   *There are not enough nursing schools and faculty members to train would-be nurses. According to ModernHealthcare.com, 78,000 applicants to bachelor and advanced-degree nursing programs were turned away in 2014.*

Shortages are more acute in some geographic areas than others. According to Vernon Lin, professor at the Cleveland Clinic Lerner College of Medicine, quoted in *The Atlantic's* "The U.S. Is Running Out of Nurses" (February 3, 2016) nursing supply is "mostly local" — i.e., nurses tend to stay in the same markets where they go to school. Fewer schools due to lack of faculty is a major cause of fewer nurses. Also, less-populated areas and poorer areas have difficulty recruiting nurses.

The shortage has serious results in that hospitals may reduce patient capacity in order to maintain proper nurse-to-patient ratios. Or the hospital may maintain purpose-specific nursing teams that can be sent wherever they are needed in the facility. Or the hospital may elect to incentivize nurses to work extra shifts, or to employ travel nurses, i.e., nurses who move from place to place on temporary assignment. All of these strategies cost the hospital money and/or place additional burdens on staff.

Hospitals that elect to handle nursing shortages by overutilization of existing staff are finding that too many patients per nurse leads to overwork and burnout. It also creates a situation in which there is a greater possibility of error. According to Professor Lin, "Past research has found links between insufficient nursing staffing and higher rates of hospital readmission and patient mortality. Higher patient loads are also linked to higher rates of nurse turnover, which can be costly, disruptive, and potentially harmful to patient safety."

Exposure To Diseases & Hazardous Chemicals

By the nature of duties that require them to work close to and come into contact with patients, nurses are regularly exposed to disease. The healthiest nurse can catch patient diseases, and hospital protocols are not always adequate to prevent the possibility.

It's difficult, in fact, to know when special protocols are necessary. If patients aren't candid about areas to which they have traveled and/or conditions to which they've been exposed, the hospital may have no idea of the need for extraordinary precautions. Even when hospitals know precautions are necessary, they may not always be ready to provide the best training and protective gear, and in the case of some diseases, there is no absolutely certain way to protect nurses from risk.

Probably the best-publicized examples of nurses contracting infectious diseases relate to the 2014 Ebola outbreak. According to the CDC, Ebola is "a rare and deadly disease caused by infection with one of the Ebola virus species." Ebola symptoms include, among other things, diarrhea, vomiting, and external bleeding, which means that caregivers may find it difficult to avoid contact with body fluids. Because Ebola is spread through direct contact with Ebola victims or objects contaminated with the body fluids of Ebola victims, elaborate safeguards were developed to protect health-care personnel who treated them. In spite of this, nurses in Madrid (Spain), Dallas (Texas, USA), Abuja (Nigeria), and Kenema (Sierra Leone) contracted the disease. Some became ill or died after being exposed to victims who had not been diagnosed, which meant that the nurses did not know to wear protective gear or follow special protocols at the time they treated the victim. Others who were following protocols and wearing protective gear say that the protocols were inconsistent or inadequate and the gear insufficient. At that time, there was no 100%-effective vaccine, so there was no sure-fire way to protect nurses and other professionals against Ebola.

As risky as situations like the Ebola outbreak may be for some nurses, hazardous chemicals may pose a greater long-term threat to all nurses. Even the latex gloves worn to protect hands can result in allergy and contact dermatitis. As for chemicals, during a typical workday, nurses are exposed to dozens of chemicals, drugs, and other potentially toxic agents or processes, many of which — according to the Environmental Working Group (EWG) — "are never tested for safety." While the exposure period for patients is brief, nurses regularly absorb minute fractions of everything they handle. The impact on nurse health of this ongoing exposure was surveyed in 2007 by EWG and Health Care Without Harm (HCWH), in collaboration with the ANA and the Environmental Health Education Center of the University of Maryland's School of Nursing. In this online survey, 1,552 nurses from across the U.S. — 80% of them registered nurses — provided information not only about their health but also that of their children in relation to eleven different common health-care hazards. This online survey revealed that exposure to sterilizing chemicals, hospital-housekeeping cleaners, residues from drug preparation, radiation, etc., led to increased rates of asthma, miscarriage, and certain cancers among nurses, and their children had increased rates of cancers and birth defects.

Other factors relating to toxic-chemical use include (1) the duration of exposure and (2) the lack of knowledge as to how the *combination* of the chemicals to which nurses are exposed may increase the risk of health problems.

Workplace-safety standards exist for only a handful of the hundreds of hazardous substances nurses may encounter in their work. There are, in fact, few mandatory protections for nurses relating to toxic chemicals, apart from the OSHA mandate requiring that manufacturers issue a Material Safety Data Sheet (MSDS) on each chemical they manufacture. It is then the responsibility of the employer to make these sheets accessible in either print or online form. Apart from this, it is up to hospitals and other employers of nurses to undertake voluntary protections, particularly by training nurses in how to protect themselves and by choosing to purchase safer products in order to avoid unnecessary risks for nurses and other employees

According to the 2007 survey by EWG and HCWH, 46% of nurses don't think their employers do enough to protect them from hazard, while 37% don't believe occupational health is taken seriously by their employers. Another 38% report that employer occupational health-education programs do not include information about chemical hazards.

Patient Liaison Difficulties

Since it is nurses who interact the most with patients, nurses will be the members of The Provider Universe who are most likely to be faced with patients who are unhappy, confused, frustrated, angry, or just plain clueless as they are confronted by some of the changes that new care-delivery models and evolving technologies will present.

Patient-centric delivery models, for example, require that providers obtain a much wider range of information from patients. This information will touch on aspects of the patient's life that he or she is likely to consider highly personal. Many patients will resist giving this information. Some will refuse. Yet, failure to acquire the information may count against the provider when it's graded by payers as to its effectiveness in the pursuit of quality and cost-control goals. Most times, it will be nurses who must persuade patients to participate, which means that it will be nurses who bear the brunt of patient hostility.

Evolving technologies will present even more specific challenges. In the broader community, there remains a suspicion, for example, of DNA testing, yet the genetics and genomic testing required for the personalized diagnostics and treatment plans of precision medicine requires that patients give permission for DNA testing. Explaining the necessity for the testing and how the results will be used will fall to the nurse, who may encounter deep-seated patient paranoia difficult to overcome even though such testing makes it possible for the provider to give the patient better care. Again, the provider may be penalized by payers for failure to administer such tests and to diagnose and treat patients according to the information that the results contain.

Probably one of the most-interesting challenges will relate to the use of biometrics for access to treatment. The use of this technology will greatly improve security and reduce fraud, so in one form or another it is almost certain to be on the near horizon for hospitals, physician offices, and other health-care facilities. There are, however, many patients who will resent being made to surrender one or more biometric identifiers in order to get access to care. As with DNA needed for genetics/genomics testing, there is in the wider community a sense that offering up for identification purposes one's physiological characteristics - fingerprints, facial features, DNA, palm prints, iris pattern, and the like - is akin to being lined up against a booking wall in a police station for a mug shot. When it's a health-care provider getting or using biometric identifiers, it will in most cases be a nurse who must explain why in a way that's acceptable to the patient.

Even after the nurse has persuaded the patient to cooperate, the patient may remain resentful or confused and not be in the mood to listen to other communication from the nurse or other staffers.

As we've seen, in order to perform at peak potential in the evolving health-care landscape, nurses must become "super communicators," but there's a problem that will be difficult to resolve. With increasing frequency, nurses do not speak the language of the patient. The Bureau of the Census reported in 2015 that over 350 languages are spoken in the fifteen largest metropolitan areas in the U.S. In the New York City metropolitan area, for example, at least 192 languages are spoken at home, and 38% of the population age five and over speak a language other than English at home. In Los Angeles, the numbers are 185 languages and 54%; in Chicago, 153 languages and 29%; in Dallas, 156 languages, and 30%; in Philadelphia, 146 languages and 15%; etc., etc., etc.

This is an issue for both doctors and nurses, most of whom have language skills limited to English and perhaps one or two other languages widely taught in the U.S., such as Spanish, French, German, Japanese, Italian, or Chinese.

Most large urban hospitals will have personnel on hand capable of translating at least some of the languages most common in the immediate area, but less-used languages can pose a quandary. When doctors are interviewing and diagnosing patients whose language they do not speak, they may have access to special translation facilities in addition to apps like Universal Doctor Speaker, but nurses in ongoing care situations may not enjoy this access and must instead rely on phrasebooks or apps, which can be awkward to use when the nurse is attempting to communicate with a patient in real time, especially if the patient is scared, in pain, angry, or under the influence of medication.

Because much nurse interaction with patients relies on the spoken word, this creates problems for both nurse and patient that can lead to errors or, at least, frustration on both sides, as well as wasted time and effort. It might even lead to or exacerbate workplace violence.

Workplace Violence

Workplace violence includes threats, assault, and/or any other behavior that creates an unsafe or threatening working environment. Studies show that the most-common sources of workplace violence in the health-care environment are:

> ◊ *Disturbed individuals in hospital emergency departments and in mental-health facilities*

◊   *Mentally incompetent elderly patients in hospital wards, nursing homes, and rehabilitation centers*

◊   *Hospital patients, their visitors, and family members who become angry at the hospital or its personnel — a particular problem with patients, visitors, and family members with a history of violent behavior*

It seems inherently contradictory to think of nurses in connection with workplace violence, for theirs is a caring occupation generally appreciated by those whose best interests they serve. At the same time, in today's more-impersonal and cost-driven environment, frustration levels are increasing among patients, patient families, and health-care co-workers (including doctors and other nurses). This leads to what some fear is becoming an epidemic of workplace violence that affects everyone who works in hospitals, particularly nurses.

Why are nurses so exposed to workplace violence?

This is a complex situation. According to *The Online Journal of Issues in Nursing: A Scholarly Journal of the American Nurses Association,* it's an issue that's complicated by two seemingly contradictory attitudes: (1) a health-care culture resistant to the idea that nurses are vulnerable to patient-related violence; and (2) the profession's acceptance that a certain amount of violence is part of the job. There is a particular problem with the latter in hospital emergency rooms where, according to a 2014 article in *Journal of Emergency Nursing,* there is an "underlying cultural acceptance" of violence.

In a way, the attitude dichotomy makes sense. On the one hand, the reasoning goes, nurses exist to help patients who are ill and in need of their care. Why would patients wish to hurt the very person who is helping them? At the same time, nurses, especially experienced nurses, understand that patients and their families are in a stressful situation that is often accompanied by fear, dread, and/or pain. Also, patients may be medicated in a way that affects their ability to comprehend what's happening or to respect normal inhibitors of behavior. It is understandable that nurses quickly develop coping mechanisms and get into the habit of being overly tolerant of patient behaviors that would not be considered acceptable in other circumstances or by other occupations.

When assessed objectively, the hospital environment in which most nurses work offers a perfect setting for violence in that:

◊   *Patients are told, implicitly or explicitly, that the hospital and its staff exist to serve them, to keep them comfortable and help them get well.*

◊   *When patients aren't comfortable, for whatever reason, and/or don't think they are benefiting from their care, they and their families and friends tend to become frustrated and even angry.*

◊   *Some patients and/or their friends and family members have a history of assault and so are predisposed to violent behavior toward others. This violent history is often unsuspected by hospital personnel.*

◊   *Patients, particularly those in psychiatric hospitals, may be momentarily or permanently incapable of maintaining appropriate behavior, due to either their condition and/or medication.*

◊   *Nurses are the hospital employees with whom patients and their families and friends most often interact, and so they are the obvious, readily accessible target for hostility.*

◊   *Security in the form of uniformed, armed guards is often minimal in most hospitals and, once a would-be malefactor is within the hospital proper, perceptibly non-existent.*

◊   *Not all hospitals have surveillance cameras and even those that do may conceal their presence so that would-be malefactors do not realize their actions may be taped.*

◊   *Ambulatory patients are encouraged to move around hospital halls in order to reduce the likelihood of their developing circulatory problems, and there is sometimes little supervision of where they go or what they do. Families and friends of patients are often allowed to come and go at will without observation by hospital personnel.*

◊   *Floor-plan layouts provide private areas in which those disposed toward violence can act out without witnesses.*

◊   *Many hospitals lack a strong violence-prevention program or even protective regulations and guidelines.*

◊   *In some work situations, not only are nurses inadequately trained in how to avoid and/or handle violence, but they are often blamed when it occurs, the thinking being that "the nurse must have done something wrong" that contributed to the development or escalation of the violent situation.*

◊   *In organizational settings where there is a culture of blame, nurses often do not report violence. This allows for the development of a cumulative impact on both individual nurses and the culture.*

◊   *Workplace violence, or its threat, contributes to nurse burnout.*

How common is violence? According to a 2014 article in *Scientific American*, almost 80% of nurses reported being attacked on the job within the past year.

Not all inappropriate behavior originates with patients and their visitors, however. Bullying among nurses is common enough that in 2008 the Center for American Nurses issued a position statement entitled "Lateral Violence and Bullying in the Workplace."

Bullying by co-workers is a special problem because there are inadequate systems in most hospitals to handle bullying, even when reported. Bullying seems to be accepted by many nurses as part of the job. The hospital environment plays a role as well when hospital administrators use fear rather than respect as a management style. Above all, many nurses claim, high workloads lead aggressive individuals unable to handle pressure-filled situations to manifest their frustration in the mistreatment of co-workers.

It is encouraging that some states have increased penalties for attacks on nurses, also that the National Institute for Occupational Safety and Health (NIOSH) is awarding grants for the development of violence-prevention programs aimed at health-care workplaces. Also, some hospitals develop extensive awareness and training programs.

Lack Of Adequate Policies For Guidance In Real-World Issues

Nurses point out that hospital policies do not always keep up with what's going on technologically or socially. Policies that lag behind real-world events leave nurses in the front lines, exposed, suspecting that they'll be faulted whatever they do.

Specific needs can vary from place to place, but situations that could pose special problems for nurses include (1) the care of protesters, (2) responding to questions relating to hospital closures or service restrictions, (3) treatment for in-the-news criminals accompanied by police or armed officers of the court, (4) patients who are celebrities, (5) staff priorities relating to new technologies, (6) handling patient or press inquiries regarding recent adverse publicity relating to the hospital or physician practice, (7) the use and misuse of social media, etc.

Nurses, by and large, are very good at what they do. Unfortunately, that doesn't necessarily include mindreading. It's up to hospitals to give nurses sensible guidelines for handling these kinds of issues.

Lack Of Respect In Relation To Responsibilities

In spite of the multiple responsibilities they assume in today's health-care environment, many nurses feel they get little respect from patients, co-workers, administrators, and doctors.

There are various reasons for this. Some of it is cultural — nurses on TV shows and in movies are often portrayed as silly layabouts or sexy predators who are out to "get" a doctor, with their patients no more than humorous props. Also, the general lack of respect awarded occupations that are primarily female automatically affects nursing, which remains overwhelmingly female. Added to this is the perception that people who elect to care for others are somehow lacking in competitive drive, which is what society values most nowadays.

Some of the lack of respect relates to the relatively invisible presence practiced by traditional nurses on the assumption that it is not the role of the nurse to put herself forward but rather to support the doctor and the patient. "I'm not there to show off," one nurse agrees. "I'm there to do my job as efficiently as possible, make sure patients get the care they need and do what I can to make them more comfortable. My goal is simply to get the patient better as quickly as possible."

Some nurses say that too-high patient-to-nurse ratios are a culprit in undermining the respect they deserve. The practice, they claim, makes it impossible for them to provide the level of care and advocacy that hospitalized patients need, a lack for which the nurses are blamed and not the budget cutters at their institution who have slashed staff numbers.

Doctors are often dismissive of nurses in front of patients and other staff, the lack of respect deriving from the fact that — better educated, better paid, better depicted in media — they are the stars of the show. Doctors who act in this way negatively influence the attitudes of patients and other staffers toward nurses. If the doctor treats nurses like nonentities, then that is how they tend to appear to others involved in the health-care process.

Hospitals may demonstrate a lack of respect by their unrealistic expectations, inadequate concern for nurse safety and health, and training that lags needs.

Worst of all, however, is that patients, employers, and co-workers often seem to place no particular value on what a nurse does.

Whatever lies behind the lack of respect accorded nurses, it seems to be a primary cause of burnout. "I have dedicated my life to this profession," one nurse told me. "I know my contribution matters, but sometimes it seems as if I'm the only one who does. That makes it even harder to accept a continually increasing workload and all the hassle that comes with it."

Expansion Of Nursing Skill Sets

There are essentially two areas that will demand the expansion of skill sets: changing care-delivery systems; and evolving technologies.

Patient-centric care-delivery systems, like PCMHs, require not only frequent communication with patients, but also communication tailored very specifically to the patient's (1) need for information or motivation and (2) ability to understand. Since it is probably nurses who will be doing much of this communication, in both hospital and other settings, theirs will inevitably be the profession inherently charged with working out many of the issues that are bound to arise for both providers and patients as these new care-delivery models move from experiment to novelty to everyday reality.

Evolving technologies pose an additional challenge. Here, communication remains critical, but the primary consideration is the need to remain up to date with changes in diagnostics, surgical techniques and devices, therapies, disease management, health-data acquisition, patient and provider access to records, and electronic health records. RNs, particularly APRNs, have always been well educated before being licensed, and then acquired more knowledge primarily through work experience; now they must view that initial educational exposure as only the beginning. Genome sequencing and genetics, augmented reality, behavior-change motivators, wearable health-data sensors, real-time diagnostics, nanorobotics, optogenetics, and biometrics are some of the technologies with which RNs and APRNs must become familiar. Familiarity with advances in these areas is necessary in order to remain valuable in a team capable of delivering quality care to patients in a cost-effective way.

As nurses deal with the new challenges facing the profession, their traditional skills of empathy, listening, and the ability to provide ongoing patient education and support will be critical. Some of the changes, however, require an expansion of the abilities traditionally associated with nursing. Three new skill sets, according to *Online Journal*, will also be necessary:

> ◊   *Nurses must become computer-adept, able to use with speed and efficiency (1) technology like email and telemedicine to share information and (2) devices like 3D printers as part of treatment processes.*

> ◊   *Nurses must acquire research skills and the ability to summarize and disseminate the information they've acquired.*

> ◊   *Nurses must understand and know how to use genomics/genetics in nursing, with a particular focus on the ethics involved.*

Many nurses are drawn to the field by a genuine wish to help those most in need of help. Once, that involved intensive amounts of interpersonal interaction with patients, a certain amount of recordkeeping, and the ability to work well with physicians, technicians, and others serving patient needs. Now, nurses must become highly skilled in communicating difficult issues and remaining up to date with new diagnostic and treatment technologies even as they retain their capacity for empathy and patient support, as well as their cooperative spirit when dealing with co-workers. It's a tricky balancing act. It's also an act that fails to get nurses the applause their efforts deserve. "It's like they want me to become this new kind of nurse, but they want to treat me the way they always have," one nurse told me. "And I'm getting fed up with it."

The Emerging Nurse Persona

Traditionally, nursing has been viewed as a profession whose members voluntarily offer their intelligence, capabilities, and commitment in the service of the greater good. That view continues to be accurate. It would be difficult to design a job description that incorporates wider scope for invaluable activity as, in collaboration with physicians and other medical-team members, the nurse brings both comfort and expert care to patients.

At the same time, the idea of "nurse as handmaiden to the doctor" is increasingly passé. The quiet, self-effacing professional whose presentation has tended to make her blend into the background environment will find herself increasingly assuming a more-assertive role.

A combination of circumstances is responsible for this shift. As physicians spend less time with patients, it is the nurse who provides much of the information and reassurance that would once have been the MD's province. As emerging care-delivery models require more information from patients, it is the nurse who will be responsible for obtaining much of it. As these same models require increased patient access to the care process, it is the nurse who will almost certainly facilitate that access. As technology becomes increasingly complex, requiring greater cooperation from patients in the gathering of samples, it is the nurse who will explain the necessity, neutralize patient resistance, and implement the process.

Of necessity, the emerging nurse persona will incorporate patient interaction of a sort that requires nurses to shift more obviously into "expert mode" with a professional assurance that will give patients confidence the nurse is now as much an authority figure as a symbol of service. This should in no way undermine the patient perception of the compassionate nurse but will add another layer to the perception.

To support this emerging persona, nurses must be willing to assume a fully collaborative role in the physician-nurse team, present their performance and their persons in a style that will help patients recognize and accept their authority, and take every opportunity offered for ongoing education.

From Florence Nightingale To Technician With A Heart

Nursing is, in the best possible sense of the term, a noble profession. This is a job that makes a real difference. That's something that few of us can say with confidence about the work that we do, but nurses affect our very lives when we are most vulnerable.

Nurses provide not only expertise but also physical and mental comforting just when we need it to get through what is possibly the most-stressful situation we'll ever have to endure. At their best, they are unsung angels. On even an average day, they are courteous and competent. And they help not only the patients in their charge but also the families and friends of those patients.

Just as significantly, nursing has always been capable of bringing great satisfaction to those who practice it. Much of that satisfaction was tied up with the interpersonal aspects of the job. Today and even more so tomorrow, the duties of the job include at least as much interaction with processes and the technologies that support them as with patients; and the ways in which technological advances will affect nursing are as yet only partly glimpsed.

It's fair to say, however, that all of us, beneficiaries at one time or another of nursing competence and dedication, must hope that a proper balance is struck between personal empathy and technological expertise. If hospitals are the liners of health care with doctors as their captains, nurses are the navigators, charting for patients an increasingly complicated course in a turbulent sea.

Chapter Twenty-One.

Morphing Roles In The Provider Universe

Even as specific educational and experience-related credentials are increasingly required to work in The Provider Universe, the roles of these highly qualified professionals are shifting.

Summary Of Issues Relating To Morphing Roles

Here are some of the issues relating to morphing roles:

◊ *Technology as driver*

◊ *Blurring of occupational lines*

◊ *Morphing roles as competitive advantage*

Technology As Driver

Traditionally, physicians practiced medicine, and all the other medical occupations supported them. In such an environment, physicians and their staffs used technology to support the doctor's intelligence, training, experience, and intuition as he (only occasionally a "she" in the traditional environment) diagnosed and treated patients.

The importance of technology as support mechanism has grown to a point where it is becoming a driver of "what happens next" and all the occupations involved in the delivery of health care, including doctors, are being forced to re-shape their approach to accommodate this devourer of traditional roles.

Here's a sampling of some of the ways in which technology, in one form or another, has changed or will soon change how things are done in The Provider Universe:

◊ *Patients will make appointments and sign in differently, and will no longer have to repeat their medical histories for each provider they visit. They will have access to their medical records online 24/7.*

◊ *Providers will rely less on heuristics (i.e., diagnosis by experience and intuition) and more on the use of decision-support software and genetics/genomics (heredity/DNA sequencing) to diagnose and treat health issues with a precision capable of making each patient intervention unique.*

◊　*Payers will have more protection against claims fraud and will also have the mechanisms needed to steer policyholders away from lower-quality providers and unproven treatments and toward better providers and proven treatments, thus saving the payer more money in the long run.*

◊　*Payers and providers will be able — by means of "smart tattoos," pills that can transmit information, and implanted sensors — to track patient compliance with treatment plans.*

The above is just the tip of the iceberg. There is no part of the health-care process that will not be affected to some extent by evolving technologies.

Blurring Of Occupational Lines

Ironically, even as requirements to perform in one medical occupation or another become more extensive and specific, thus increasing the number of medical specialties, evolving technologies will begin to devalue detailed knowledge that is readily available via online databases and decision-support software. Instead of rewarding a relatively static skill set, the coming medical environment will demand that all health-care occupations be capable of:

◊　*Efficient accessing of the latest information as to best practices*

◊　*A high level of interpretation and assimilation of information*

◊　*Excellent communications skills*

Just as critical will be the need for all professionals to be capable of outstanding teamwork that focuses on patient care rather than individual turfs.

Other factors that will accelerate the blurring of occupational lines include:

◊　*Technology as driver of diagnostic/treatment process (see above)*

◊　*The movement to treat patients in nontraditional settings by medical practitioners other than MDs*

◊　*The need for flexibility and versatility in a cost- and quality-conscious environment undergoing continual change*

◊　*The growing importance of patient communications in the Patient-Centered Medical Home (PCMH), communications that typically will be handled by nurses or other staffers rather than MDs*

In combination, these factors will create unintended outcomes, specifically situations in which staffers other than the physician may assume a leadership role in one part or another of medical interventions. This suggests that medical personnel, including physicians, would benefit from training in how to use the new technologies to improve patient care without triggering intraoccupational conflict and turf struggles.

Morphing Roles As Competitive Advantage

Theoretically, all providers can learn how to use medical advances and have access to technological improvements. That knowledge and access, in fact, will become given, something that patients take for granted.

This means that the only reliable competitive advantage — in a marketplace where competition for reimbursement is largely based on patient outcomes and satisfaction — lies in the human factor. It will still matter that MDs, NPs, PAs, and other staffers are technically proficient, but it will matter just as much that they deliver the kind of care that patients *perceive* to be valuable.

This may well mean that providers ambitious to gain the greatest reimbursement advantage will return to a more-personal approach to medical interventions, whichever occupation is interacting with the patient at any given time — more time spent explaining things, more effort exerted in responding to patient concerns, more of everything that will make patients feel better about the care they receive. It matters to outcomes that patients recognize their care as exceptional, as that makes them more likely to do their part to get well and stay well by following doctor's orders and making health-enhancing lifestyle changes.

I recall when my grandmother had cataract surgery years ago that required a hospital stay, a situation that had almost paralyzed her with fear, the doctor sat with her the day before the surgery, listening to her concerns, holding her hand, and murmuring encouragement. The day after the surgery, I arrived to find a LPN at her bedside, softly singing her favorite hymn. The culture in that small, privately owned hospital seemed to be totally patient-focused, and even though my grandmother's medical outcome was not outstanding by today's standards, she never stopped bragging about the excellent care she'd received and how wonderful the hospital was.

We'll never return to those days, but making medicine feel more personal again could become a powerful competitive device that can be employed by every member of the care team. History and human nature suggest that it could be the human factor that makes the difference in the end.

PART THREE.
PATIENTS IN THE CHANGING PROVIDER UNIVERSE

Chapter Twenty-Two.

What The Changing Provider Universe Means for Patients

Everything that's happening in The Provider Universe affects patients to one degree or another. Because so much of what shapes The Provider Universe — and thus the experience of the patients who enter it — is political in origin and U.S. politics are subject to influences that are difficult to anticipate or sometimes make sense of, the analysis that follows is not so much a prediction as a consideration of the outcomes that logic suggests could follow trends that have already emerged, are in the works, or appear likely given medical advances, technological evolution, and the need to control costs and improve outcomes.

Summary Of What Will Be Affected By Change

We'll look at:

◊   *What in the patient experience will be affected by change*

◊   *Drivers for change*

◊   *What this might mean for a typical health episode*

◊   *Tradeoffs for patients*

◊   *An end to aging or just a delay of the inevitable?*

◊   *Outlook - The dream and what probably lies ahead for patients*

Let me emphasize again that these are not predictions per se, but an educated guess based on current trends.

What In The Patient Experience Will Be Affected

Changes in The Provider Universe affect, or will affect, the very basics of health care, including:

◊   *A patient's right to access his or her own health records*

◊   *Who can access health care and how*

◊   *Where, how, and when health care is delivered*

◊   *What Medicare, insurance companies, and employers self-insured as to employee health care will pay for and what will become the responsibility of the patient*

◊   *How much responsibility patients will be expected to assume for the management of their health*

The degree to which each aspect of health care will be affected will depend on a combination of drivers.

Drivers For Change In Patient Care

Here are some of the drivers and how they'll affect patient care:

◊   *Medical advances and technological developments — particularly the use of genetics/genomics (heredity/DNA sequencing in plain English) — will make available a wider range of diagnostic and treatment tools, enabling precision medicine, that is, care that is targeted very specifically to a particular patient and his or her health issue. This should result in more-successful patient outcomes.*

◊   *There will be less-painful and intrusive diagnostic tests, like a test for blood proteins linked to heart disease that may substitute for diagnostic angiograms. Or how about tattoos that can monitor blood glucose without a finger prick?*

◊   *Nanorobots will perform less-intrusive and more-targeted surgeries, making possible not only better outcomes but also faster recovery times.*

◊   *Physicians will use decision-support software to verify diagnosis and determine "best practices" for a patient's specific condition and situation. This will make error less likely and should lead to better outcomes and faster recovery.*

◊   *Hospitals will become more careful about hygiene and more determined to avoid medical error, as their reimbursement from payers will be increasingly reduced in relation to these factors. This should result in safer hospital stays for patients.*

◊   *The use of bioink based on the patient's own body chemistry in medical 3D printing to generate organs for transplant will make possible (1) a greater number of organ transplants without any waiting period and (2) transplants less likely to be rejected by the patient's body. This will increase longevity for patients needing transplants and reduce the need for rejection treatments or even repeated transplants.*

◊ *Optogenetics therapy holds the promise of ending the need to take stimulants, painkillers, and tranquilizers. This will not only be healthier for patients, but will also reduce drug abuse and addiction.*

◊ *Escalating drug costs will result in more pharmaceuticals being removed or omitted from insurance-company formularies, and many patients, insured or not, will elect not to continue taking the drugs because they can't afford to.*

◊ *The ability via eHealth apps and sensor devices to self-monitor and even to send information relating to diet, exercise, blood pressure, heart rate, etc., to providers or payers will (1) encourage patients to follow doctor's orders and (2) enable providers and payers to determine the degree to which the patient is adhering to treatment plans.*

◊ *The growing ability of providers to use medical advances and new technologies to keep patients alive indefinitely, even if essentially non-functioning, will encourage more patients who do not want this degree of care to write living wills stipulating their wishes as to treatment and designating health-care executors.*

◊ *Access by patients to online medical information, hospital safety grades, and provider reviews will (1) affect their choice of providers and opinion toward diagnoses and treatment plans and (2) enable them to leave their own comments and/or reviews.*

◊ *The satisfaction surveys that patients complete following treatment will play a role of increasing importance in the way in which providers are reimbursed for care. This will make providers attempt to deliver care so that patients not only receive quality but also recognize it.*

◊ *The consolidation of physician practices, hospital systems, health-insurance companies, and pharmaceutical companies will limit patient choices as to providers, as will narrow networks.*

◊ *Health-care fraud will prompt the introduction of more-stringent proof-of-identity requirements, which will lead providers to adopt biometric identifiers at sign-in as a precondition for care.*

◊ Patient-centric care-delivery models like Patient-Centered Medical Homes (PCMHs) will be the equivalent of the bar "where everyone knows your name" or at least has access to your EHRs 24/7 and a vested financial interest in keeping you healthy or returning you to health as quickly and effectively as possible.

◊ PCMHs will also require that providers obtain information from patients about their lifestyles and preferences as to health care. Some of this information will be highly personal, and many patients will resist providing it, especially if they have doubts about the ability of HIPAA to keep the information private from family members and employers.

◊ PCMHs will (1) give patients and, in some instances, their families more input into the care process and (2) require greater patient cooperation with treatment plans.

◊ The determination of Medicare and other payers to switch from fee-for-service to fee-for-performance will encourage providers to (1) focus on quality rather than quantity of care and (2) demand greater accountability from patients as to self-management of health. Physicians may be tempted to turn away patients who do not follow treatment plans or in other ways undermine care outcomes because poor outcomes will reduce their rate of reimbursement. While some physicians consider it inappropriate to refuse to treat patients due to their lifestyle choices, it is evidently not illegal unless the refusal is based on ethnic, racial, or religious reasons.

◊ Electronic health records (EHRs), once fully in place, will eliminate duplicative treatment and other errors even as they enable patients and their health-care providers to access health histories 24/7.

◊ Medical-identity fraud will have increased significance once EHRs are fully operational because any information tied to the "illegal" patient's use of a health plan — which is usually the point of stealing such information — will be entered into the "legal" individual's record, thus corrupting its integrity and undermining its usefulness as an aid to diagnosis and treatment.

◊ The growing sophistication of hackers will force hospitals, medical practices, insurance companies, and other entities involved in the provision of care or its payment to institute more-stringent security measures, which should mean greater protection for patient information and less likelihood of medical-identity fraud.

◊   *Escalating profit expectations and the growing demand for health-care services in relation to supply will keep health care expensive. This will encourage employers to shift more of the cost to employees in the form of higher co-pays and deductibles and will also mean an ongoing increase in health-insurance premiums.*

◊   *Even as some patients give up a degree of choice in order to stay within insurance-plan care networks and thus save money, other patients will be willing to pay extra to sign up with concierge practices that allow them extra time with the doctor.*

◊   *As even insured patients have to pay more for care and are pressured to assume accountability for self-management, they will become more demanding in their expectations of a user-friendly and effective health-care system.*

Singly and in combination, these drivers will result in a restructuring of the priorities of both patients and the providers who treat them. There should be more transparency from every provider involved in patient treatment as to:

◊   *What is to be done*

◊   *Why it is being done*

◊   *What it will cost*

◊   *Who will pay*

◊   *The likely outcome*

There will be greater awareness on the part of patients that they must:

◊   *Participate in the making of treatment plans*

◊   *Accept more responsibility for adhering to treatment plans and engaging in preventive care*

◊   *Understand that there may be penalties for ignoring doctor's orders and maintaining unhealthy habits*

Patient Tradeoffs

It's likely that the matter of (1) choice vs. cost and (2) personal privacy vs. improved care due to precision medicine will be a source of political and ethical contention, particularly once patients realize the implications.

Many patients will dislike the growing expectation that they accept more accountability for their health management, even though this enhances their likelihood of living longer in better physical and mental condition and gives them greater input into treatment options.

Patients will particularly resist pressure from insurance companies, employers who pay some or all of health costs, and providers to change lifestyle habits that produce risk factors for serious disease. It's possible, however, that the knowledge made possible by some of the processes associated with precision medicine will produce information that allows patients to recognize without doubt certain habits as causes of diseases that most people would do almost anything to avoid.

Chapter Twenty-Three.

A Typical Health Episode Today & Tomorrow

The changes in The Provider Universe will, by and large, appear gradually, oftentimes more a matter of degree than an abrupt transformation. Over time, however, they will have a basic impact on how patient care is handled. Let's take a look at the handling of a common health event to see what's likely to change.

Jane's Health Event

Jane, an accountant in a large consulting firm, is a daily jogger. One day, after her usual run, she feels an acute pain in her knee. She tries icing it, wrapping it in an elastic bandage, and resting it, but the pain persists. She knows she needs medical care. She considers going to the urgent-care center she used when she sprained her wrist, but suspects her knee requires more-intensive treatment than is available there. Below we'll compare how medical intervention would be handled today by many providers and is likely to be handled the day after tomorrow.

Medical Intervention Today

◊ *Jane calls or visits the office of her primary-care physician to get his referral to an orthopedist.*

◊ *At the orthopedist's, Jane presents the identification card issued by the company that insures her employer's workforce.*

◊ *Jane signs a form stating that she will be responsible for any co-pays, deductibles, and expenses not covered by her plan. Depending on the office, she will be asked for a payment toward co-pays either upfront or before she leaves the office. Later, she will be billed for anything else her insurance plan doesn't pay.*

◊ *A nurse takes her blood pressure, then weighs her and notes the result in her file, which is then taken into the examining room and handed over to the doctor who is waiting to see Jane.*

◊   The doctor examines Jane's knee and asks her questions relating specifically to the injury. Jane's responses are noted in her file by the nurse.

◊   Midway through the visit, Jane is taken down the hall to a technician, who x-rays or scans her knee. When the result is ready, the MD puts it up on a monitor and indicates the area of the problem to Jane. Nothing is broken, but there is an issue that should be addressed. She will, he tells her, need surgery, which can be performed at the nearby regional medical center. His office will make the arrangements and will call to verify time and place.

◊   As Jane's knee is swollen, indicating the possibility of inflammation, the MD gives her a shot of penicillin and says he will prescribe a painkiller but needs to determine any medication she's already taking before giving her a new prescription. She tells him she isn't taking any other medication, and he has his nurse call in a prescription to Jane's preferred pharmacy.

◊   The entire visit requires probably an hour, depending on the speed of the x-ray/scanning process. Jane's knee injury is treated as a one-off event with no attention being paid to anything other than the specific injury.

◊   Jane goes to the pharmacy, picks up the prescription, charging it to a credit card because her insurance plan does not cover prescriptions.

◊   Back at the orthopedist's, before the surgery is scheduled, the MD's office manager calls the administrator of Jane's insurance plan to make sure the surgery is covered, and then calls the hospital to schedule the date for Jane's outpatient surgery.

◊   On the day of the surgery, Jane goes to the outpatient facility of the hospital, has arthroscopic surgery, and is released that same day. The hospital bills Jane for any co-pays, deductibles, or expenses not covered by her insurance plan.

◊   The orthopedist's office schedules a follow-up appointment a week later, at which the MD examines Jane's knee, says it appears to be doing well, and schedules a follow-up appointment for the next month. When the time for the appointment arrives, Jane is unable to keep it and must call to change its time.

◊   Each time that Jane visits the orthopedist's office, she sees the MD, *and presents a credit card to cover any charges she owes.*

◊ *Jane will hear nothing further from the hospital, and once her final visit to the orthopedist is completed and she is dismissed, she will hear nothing further from the orthopedist's office.*

◊ *If, months later, Jane awakes in the middle of the night with her knee in excruciating pain, she can either go to the hospital emergency room or wait until the next morning and call the orthopedist's office for the first available appointment.*

◊ *Throughout the period of diagnosis and treatment for her knee condition, everything that's done will become part of Jane's files at the orthopedist's office and at the hospital — and she has the right to see her health record at any point during or following the care event. To see the file, she must make application to the provider in written form, according to state law. If the orthopedist and hospital have digitized their records, Jane can access them 24/7 for free via the providers' online portals.*

◊ *After questioning a couple of items, Jane pays any bills remaining from the care episode after the insurance plan has paid its share.*

◊ *As long as Jane's knee does not bother her again, this care episode is over, and Jane can relax. Her knee is better, and her insurance plan will cover any such episode should it occur again. There will be no question of penalties, cancellation, or any other insurance-related issues because she is part of a group plan.*

◊ *Any paper files relating to Jane's surgery will remain in the offices of the orthopedist and the hospital where, unless they are physically stolen or someone goes to the trouble to copy or photograph them, they will remain free from intrusion or misuse.*

Medical Intervention Tomorrow

◊ *Jane checks the app issued by her insurance plan to verify who in her geographic area is in the plan's network for an orthopedic injury, clicks the link, then makes an appointment online for an initial visit.*

◊ *At the orthopedist's, Jane passes her hand across a biometric reader, which recognizes her palm print, tying it to her EHR, which contains full details of her health history and current insurance plan.*

◊   Jane indicates the method of payment she'll use to cover what the biometric identifier has enabled the provider office to determine is the co-pay and deductible she will owe for this visit. Typically, she will specify (1) a credit or debit card, (2) automatic withdrawal from her checking account, or (3) debiting of her medical savings account.

◊   If this information is not already part of her EHR, Jane will be asked to indicate her preferred pharmacy.

◊   Jane steps upon a body scanner's platform and inserts two fingers into side-by-side sensors. Information as to her height, weight, temperature, pulse, and blood oxygen level is immediately transmitted to her EHR for review by a PA on the widescreen monitor mounted on the wall of the examination room. Her blood pressure is taken, and that information similarly entered into her EHR. The PA examines Jane's knee and inputs her answers to his questions into a laptop on the counter next to him, at which point they become part of her EHR. His questions relate not only to the specific injury, but also to new information related to lifestyle issues not already entered into her EHR that might have caused the injury or affect the treatment process, particularly diet, exercise, and personal habits such as smoking, drinking, and recreational drug use.

◊   At a certain point in the visit, as soon as the PA is sure of the afflicted area, Jane will be taken down the hall to a technician who will digitally scan her knee. The results of the scan immediately become part of Jane's EHR. The PA reads the results of the scan with Jane, then the orthopedist enters, reads the scan, looks at Jane's knee, consults Jane's EHR, asks the PA a couple of questions, and tells Jane that she needs surgery. He says that the surgery will be performed on an outpatient basis, which can be done either in this office or in the nearby regional medical facility. Jane's insurance plan, however, will pay only if the surgery is performed at the medical facility's outpatient surgical unit, so he assumes that is what she will prefer. He says she can check the office's online portal by the end of the day for details of day and time. The MD departs, on his way to see the next patient.

◊   As Jane's knee is not only hurting but swollen, the PA selects two medications from the list the decision-support software indicates are appropriate for the symptoms and diagnosis he has entered, one an antibiotic and one a painkiller. There are no conflicts with medication Jane is already taking, and so the system automatically transmits the *prescriptions to Jane's preferred pharmacy. If there had been conflict the software would have prompted the PA to select a different medication.*

◊ *The entire visit requires probably forty minutes, including time needed for the scan and waiting for the MD to appear. The information provided by Jane in the initial examination and already present in her EHR will trigger certain population health management associations and when preparing for the surgery, the MD will look at Jane not just as an individual patient but as a non-smoking 28-year-old Hispanic female, an occasional drinker, working a white-collar desk job, living in an older part of a zip code known for its cracked pavements and uneven sidewalks. As part of his preparation for surgery, the MD will consult decision-support software for access to the latest research and best practices for treatment of this kind of knee issue in a woman of Jane's age, ethnicity, occupation, etc.*

◊ *Jane goes to the pharmacy and learns that one of the prescribed medications isn't covered by her insurance plan (which covers prescriptions). The pharmacy has notified the orthopedist's office of an acceptable equivalent that is covered, and the PA has agreed. Jane's prescriptions are ready.*

◊ *Back at the orthopedist's, the process to schedule the surgery has already been completed via software interactions among Jane's insurance plan, the facility where the surgery will take place, and the office of the surgeon.*

◊ *By the time Jane gets home, she can go onto the orthopedist's online portal and print out the diagnosis she was given. She can also learn where and when surgery is to take place. The information provided not only gives her scheduling details but also stipulates the co-pay and deductible she will owe. If the proposed time frame is acceptable and she agrees with the monetary stipulations, she is to confirm the appointment via digital signature. If the information provided is not acceptable, she is to refuse the appointment and indicate a date range that will work for her and any questions she has as to costs.*

◊ *Online, Jane also researches the precise diagnosis she has been given, noting that the treatment prescribed for her condition is typical and generally effective, resulting in a recovery period of from six weeks to three months. She also checks the safety grade for the facility where the surgery is to be performed and finds it acceptable.*

◊   On the day of the surgery, Jane goes to the regional medical center's outpatient surgery facility, does the biometric scan, which ties her to her insurance plan, her health history, and the diagnostics and treatment plan tied to this particular intervention, has nanorobotic surgery to repair torn ligaments, is released a few hours later and goes home.

◊   The orthopedist's office schedules a follow-up appointment a week later, at which the PA examines Jane's knee, says it appears to be doing well, and schedules a follow-up appointment for the next month. When the time for the appointment arrives, Jane is unable to keep it because she is unexpectedly out of town on business. Rather than cancel, she goes onto the orthopedist's online portal and requests a telemedicine session. Within an hour, she is signaled that she has a communication in the online portal. When she goes online, she receives an address and time for a telemedicine visit in a nearby medical center. At the telemedicine center, Jane's palm is scanned and the $100 co-pay is automatically debited against Jane's preferred payment method before the telemedicine visit begins.

◊   When Jane next visits the orthopedist's office in person, she may be surprised to find a new MD is in charge of her case because the MD who did the surgery is no longer part of that practice, but has moved out of town to a practice in a nearby state. The payment method she indicated at her first visit is debited for her share of the cost of the visit.

◊   At some point following the surgery, Jane will receive a questionnaire from either the hospital or the insurance plan asking her to assess the quality of the care she received. If she does not complete this right away, she will be asked again. Jane completes the questionnaire carefully because she knows that her answers will affect the provider's reimbursement from her insurance plan. If Jane never completes the questionnaire, she may be penalized by her insurance plan.

◊   If, months later, Jane awakes in the middle of the night with her knee in excruciating pain, she can go at once to a 24/7 urgent-care center or, since her orthopedist is part of a PCMH, she has a phone number she can call at any hour to share her concerns and get rapid counsel as to what to do.

◊   Throughout the period of diagnosis and treatment for her knee condition, everything that's done will become part of Jane's EHR — which she has the right to see online 24/7 at any point during or following the care event. If, during the course of the knee treatment, Jane *goes to another medical provider for an unrelated condition, the information generated there will immediately become part of Jane's EHR and may affect subsequent decisions regarding the knee treatment.*

◊ *By the time Jane has completed her last appointment with the orthopedist, there are no bills left to be paid, as all of the providers involved automatically debited Jane's preferred payment method for her share of costs.*

◊ *Jane's health plan is through her employer, but it is written in several tiers relating to employees hitting health targets. Those who hit them get discounts off the employee share of premiums. Jane may have a few nervous moments as she contemplates what the claims filed in connection with her knee injury might do to her share of premiums, but the insurance company notifies her that her coverage will be continued in the same tier with no increase in her share of premiums because the information periodically transmitted to them from her health sensor (heart rate, blood pressure, alcohol intake, smoking habits, diet, exercise, etc.) shows that she's been following a healthy regimen well within the orthopedist's guidelines. Also, the weigh-in at her physician's office showed that her weight remains well within the acceptable BMI (body mass index). Also, the company's risk calculator indicates that, given Jane's age and physical condition, the health benefits of jogging compensate for the fact that participation in the activity was the cause of her injury.*

◊ *At some point after Jane's knee issue is resolved — perhaps years later — she may receive an email from her insurance plan stating that its patient database has been hacked and it's possible that some or all of Jane's information has been accessed. She will be advised to go online and get further information from the IT group dealing with the issue. At that point, she will either be reassured, or she will be told to change her online-portal password, user ID, etc., and given free access to a credit-monitoring service that has been retained to assist customers needing to keep an eye on their financial identity due to the increased risk for fraud.*

Primary Differences Between Today & Tomorrow

If current trends continue, tomorrow's health intervention will be less personal, more personalized, and more user-friendly. Jane will use HIT to determine the provider her health plan recommends, book the appointment, and sign in. The biometric identifier she provides at sign-in will drive the rest of the health intervention, given that it's tied to her insurance plan, preferred payment method, and previous health history. In the provider's office, Jane's visit will be made more accurate and briefer through the use of advanced technologies to acquire health indicators, perform diagnostic scans, assess the diagnosis, and prescribe medication. At the pharmacy, the problem with the non-covered prescription will have been resolved via computer interaction before her arrival. Meanwhile, the provider will have used HIT to schedule surgery as per the requirements of Jane's insurance plan. Back home, Jane can not only verify the details of her diagnosis online, but also check her calendar and verify agreement to the surgery as scheduled. The surgery will be less invasive and more precise, with a faster recovery. The follow-up exams will be scheduled online, and telemedicine will make it possible for Jane to keep an exam appointment when she must be out of town. Health sensors proving she maintains a lifestyle that will support ongoing knee health save her from being subjected to a premium penalty by her employer's insurance plan. All along, each time that service is provided, any money Jane owes for deductibles, co-pays, and/or noncovered expenses will have been paid, as per her directions, via (1) debiting of a credit card, (2) withdrawal from a checking account, or (3) charge against her medical savings account.

The entire process will be both more efficient and more effective. As a patient, Jane will benefit from improved diagnostics, "best practices" decision support, more-precise surgery, and more-consistent follow-up; she must also assume greater responsibility than today for doing her part to get well and stay well and to comply with provider and insurance-plan directives throughout. As an individual, Jane will enjoy greater convenience, premium savings, no monetary surprises, and shorter time frames for each stage of the process. Any sense that she has been on a medical assembly line, where her performance as well as that of her provider is graded, will probably be ameliorated by the knowledge that she has had the best care and been able to return to her usual routine well within the time frame predicted by her research into her condition.

Chapter Twenty-Four.

The Dream, The Promise & The Likely Reality

Most of the changes in The Provider Universe are the result of someone's idea of how to make things better for patient health care, a decades-in-the-works culmination of the creativity and intelligence of a lot of dedicated professionals. Correctly coordinated and properly executed, all these ideas are capable of helping us achieve not just longer life, but better life. The most-tantalizing possibility, of course, is that we remain ourselves at our physical and mental best for as long as life can be prolonged. Is this achievable? The answer is a qualified "yes" – probably (the redundancy is deliberate).

An End To Aging Or Just A Delay Of The Inevitable?

Theoretically, the rapid evolution of highly targeted, individualized therapies may mean an "end to aging" and, possibly, even a reversal of the aging process.

What's more certain is that advancing technologies will continue to inch toward the potential for an indefinite prolongation of life, whatever the overall mental or physical condition of the patient.

There are those who predict that the human body will become a mass of interchangeable parts, capable of endless repair, and that the individual's brain will be reinstalled in the repaired body or even a completely rebuilt shell.

The medical and societal costs associated with this possibility almost certainly mean that it will be available not by insurance coverage or government program but only to those able to pay for it out of pocket. For everyone else, the likelihood is that we will enjoy somewhat longer life spans during which we have the benefit of health outcomes that are outstanding when compared to those of earlier generations but that do not necessarily incorporate every possibility of the latest and greatest in patient care.

Outlook – The Dream & What Probably Lies Ahead For Patients

The dream is that a coordinated provider environment will deliver carefully calibrated attention to all Americans that will keep them well as long as possible and then will tend to their ailments in an efficient and reasonably caring manner. Along the way, all those entities involved will earn reasonable profits, and public health will improve as private health goals are met.

The reality is likely to be a system in transition for years to come. Many of the improvements will exist more in theory than in practice as providers continue to be distracted by financial, political, administrative, and information-technology challenges. Theoretically, everything they do is related in some way to the provision of better, more cost-effective care for patients, from how they organize their functions to staffing priorities to payer relations and everything in between. Most care providers would rather spend more time with patients and less time with these other aspects of The Provider Universe. The reality, however, is that activities not directly related to patients must go on.

The Bottom Line

Patients will continue to be just one of the elements to which providers must pay attention. Individual patients will have sustained, automatic clout only to the extent that their outcomes and levels of satisfaction are monitored and made part of a collective metric that shapes how delivery of medical services is prioritized and reimbursed. Otherwise, our care — as it has always — will rely on the professionalism, intelligence, talents, resources, and willingness of our providers.

In Closing

The future of American health care hesitates at some barely glimpsed, on-the-horizon intersection of provider capabilities, technological possibilities, corporate profit margins, governmental budgets, public policy, and personal responsibility. As yet, it's a hazy glimmer that will come into focus only as we decide and have the will to act upon our personal and public priorities in relation to health.

The End

APPENDICES

Appendix A.

Acronyms Used In The Book

AAMC	Association of American Medical Colleges
AAFP	American Academy of Family Physicians
AANP	American Association of Nurse Practitioners
ACA	2010 Patient Protection and Affordable Care Act (Popular Nickname: Obamacare)
ACEP	American College of Emergency Physicians
ACO	Accountable Care Organization
ACP	American College of Physicians
ADA	Americans with Disabilities Act
AHA	American Hospital Association
AHRQ	Agency for Healthcare Research and Quality
ALS	Amyotrophic lateral sclerosis, aka Lou Gehrig disease
AMA	American Medical Association
ANA	American Nurses Association
ANCC	American Nurses Credentialing Center
APHIS	Animal and Plant Health Inspection Service
APM	Alternative payment model
APRN	Advanced-practice registered nurse
ATF	American Transplant Foundation

BARDA	Biomedical Advanced Research and Development Authority
BLS	Bureau of Labor Statistics
BMI	Body mass index
BMT	Blood & Marrow Transplant
BPCI	Bundled Payment Care Improvement
CAUTI	Catheter-associated urinary tract infections
CBO	U.S. Congressional Budget Office
CDC	Centers for Disease Control and Prevention
CDER	FDA's Center for Drug Evaluation and Research
CDSS	Clinical decision support system
CFO	Chief financial officer
CHIP	Children's Health Insurance Program
CLIA	Clinical Laboratory Improvement Amendments of 1998
CMMI	Center for Medicare and Medicaid Innovation, aka CMS Innovation Center
CLABSI	Central line-associated bloodstream infections
CMS	Centers for Medicare & Medicaid Services
COBRA	Consolidated Omnibus Budget Reconciliation Act of 1985
CPOE	Computerized Provider Order Entry
CPT	Current Procedure Terminology
CT	Computed tomography
DEA	Drug Enforcement Administration
DHHS	U.S. Department of Health & Human Services
DNA	Deoxyribonucleic acid

DNDI	Drugs for Neglected Diseases Initiative
DNP	Doctor of Nursing Practice
DOJ	U.S. Department of Justice
DOL	U.S. Department of Labor
ED	Emergency department
EHR	Electronic health record
EMT	Emergency medical technician
EMTALA	Emergency Medical Treatment & Labor Act
EPA	Environmental Protection Agency
ER	Emergency room
EWG	Environmental Working Group
FACMPE	Fellow in the American College of Medical Practice
FACS	Fellow of the American College of Surgeons
FBI	Federal Bureau of Investigation
FDA	Food and Drug Administration
FTC	Federal Trade Commission
GAO	U.S. Government Accountability Office
GDP	Gross Domestic Product
HAI	Hospital-acquired infection
HERC	Healthcare Environmental Resource Center
HCAHPS and Systems	Hospital Consumer Assessment of Healthcare Providers
HCWH	Health Care Without Harm
HIPAA 1996	Health Insurance Portability and Accountability Act of

HIT	Health information technology
HLOC	Health Locus of Control
HRSA	Health Resources & Services Administration
IARC	International Agency for Research on Cancer
ICD	International Classification of Diseases
ICU	Intensive care unit
IDSA	Infectious Disease Society of America
IFHP	International Federation of Health Plans
IHME	Institute of Health Metrics and Evaluation at University of Washington
IMP	Ideal Micropractice
IOM	Institute of Medicine
IPN	International Policy Network
IQI	Inpatient quality indicator
IT	Information technology
IV	Intravenous
JAMA	*Journal of the American Medical Association*
LCME	Liaison Committee on Medical Education
LLC	Limited liability company
LLS	Leukemia & Lymphoma Society
LPN	Licensed practical nurse
LTACH	Long-term acute care hospitals
MACRA	Medicare Access and CHIP Reauthorization Act of 2015
MB&C	Medical coding and billing
MD	Doctor of Medicine

MHA	Master of Health Administration
MOC	Maintenance of certification
MRI	Magnetic resonance imaging
MRSA	Methicillin-resistant *Staphylococcus Aureus*
MS	Multiple sclerosis
NAM	National Academy of Medicine
NEJM	*New England Journal of Medicine*
NP	Nurse Practitioner
NQF	National Quality Forum
NHLBI	National Heart, Lung, and Blood Institute
NIH	National Institutes of Health
NIOSH	National Institute for Occupational Safety and Health
NMHC	Nurse-Managed Health Clinic
NP	Nurse Practitioner
OCE	U.S. Office of Congressional Ethics
OCR	U.S. Office for Civil Rights
OMB	U.S. Office of Management and Budget
OOH	Occupational Outlook Handbook
ORI	Oregon Research Institute
OSHA	Occupational Safety and Health Administration
OSTP	U.S. Office of Science and Technology Policy
OTC	Over-the-counter
PA	Physician Assistant
PA-C	Physician Assistant-Certified
PBM	Pharmacy benefit management

PCMH	Patient-Centered Medical Home
PCP	Primary care physician
PDI	Pediatric quality indicator
PFPM	Physician Focused Payment Model
PHI	Protected health information
PHM	Population health management
PhRMA	Pharmaceutical Research and Manufacturers of America
PHSO	Population health support organization
PLC	Public limited company
PQRS	Physician Quality Reporting System
PSI	Patient safety indicator
PSQH	Patient Safety & Quality Healthcare
R&D	Research and development
RN	Registered nurse
SGR	Sustainable Growth Rate
SPHHS	School of Public Health and Health Services
SRE	Serious reportable event
SSI	Surgical-site infections
THCGME	Teaching Health Center Graduate Medical Education Payment Program
UA	Urinalysis
UNC	University of North Carolina
UNOS	United Network for Organ Sharing
UPMC	University of Pittsburgh Medical Center
VCA	Vascularized composite allografts

VI	Vertical integration
VR	Virtual reality
WHO	World Health Organization
YMCA	Young Men's Christian Association

Appendix B.

Useful Online Resources: A Selection

Certification & Licensing Boards

Accreditation Council for Graduate Medical Education
http://www.acgme.org

Addiction Professionals Certification Board, Inc.
https://certbd.org

American Academy of Nurse Practitioners Certification Board
https://www.aanpcert.org

American Board for Certification in Orthotics, Prosthetics &
Pedorthics (ABCOP)
https://www.abcop.org

American Board of Addiction Medicine
https://www.abam.net/become-certified/

American Board of Allergy and Immunology (ABAI)
https://www.abai.org

American Board of Audiology (ABA)
http://www.boardofaudiology.org/board-certified-in-audiology/

American Board of Family Medicine (ABFM)
https://www.theabfm.org

American Board of Genetic Counseling, Inc. (ABGC)
http://www.abgc.net/Certification/certification.asp

American Board of Internal Medicine (ABIM)
http://www.abim.org

American Board of Medical Specialties (ABMS)
http://www.abms.org

American Board of Neurological Surgery (ABNS)
http://www.abns.org

American Board of Nuclear Medicine (ABNM)
https://www.abnm.org

American Board of Obstetrics + Gynecology (ABO+G)
https://www.abog.org

American Board of Ophthalmology (ABO)
http://abop.org

American Board of Optometry
http://americanboardofoptometry.org

American Board of Orthopaedic Surgery (ABOS)
https://www.abos.org

American Board of Otolaryngology (ABOto)
http://www.aboto.org

American Board of Pathology (ABOP)
http://www.abpath.org

American Board of Pediatrics (ABP)
https://www.abp.org

American Board of Pediatric Medicine (ABPM)
http://www.abprevmed.org

American Board of Plastic Surgery, Inc.
https://www.abplasticsurgery.org

American Board of Psychiatry and Neurology, Inc. (ABPN)
https://www.abpn.com

American Board of Radiology (ABR)
https://www.theabr.org

American Board of Surgery (ABS)
http://www.absurgery.org

American College of Medical Practice Executives (ACMPE)
http://www.mgma.com/education-certification/medical-practice-
management-certification-through

American College of Surgeons
https://www.facs.org/education/accreditation

American Medical Billing Association (AMBA)
http://www.ambanet.net/AMBA.htm

American Midwifery Certification Board (AMCB)
http://www.amcbmidwife.org

American Nurses Credentialing Center (ANCC)
http://www.nursecredentialing.org

Association of Boards of Certification (ABC)
http://www.abccert.org

*Certification Board of Cardiovascular Computed Tomography
(CBCCT)*
http://www.cccvi.org/cbcct/

*Certification Board of Infection Control and Epidemiology, Inc.
(CBIC)*
https://www.cbic.org

Certification Board of Nuclear Cardiology (CBNC)
http://www.cccvi.org/cbnc/

Federation of State Medical Boards (FSMB)
http://www.fsmb.org

Hospice Medical Director Certification Board (HMDCB)
http://www.hmdcb.org

Medical Management Institute (MMI)
http://mmiclasses.com/mmi-membership/

National Board for Certification of School Nurses (NBCSN)
http://www.nbcsn.org

National Board of Medical Examiners (NBME)
http://www.nbme.org

National Certification Board for Diabetes Educators (NCBDE)
https://www.ncbde.org

Nuclear Medicine Technology Certification Board
https://www.nmtcb.org

Pharmacy Technician Certification Board (PTCB)
https://www.ptcb.org

*The Joint Commission (accredits and certifies nearly 21,000 health-
care organizations and programs in the U.S.)*
https://www.jointcommission.org/about_us/about_the_joint_
commission_main.aspx

Government Health-Related Sites

ACOs in Your State / CMS.gov
https://www.cms.gov/medicare/medicare-fee-for-service-payment/
sharedsavingsprogram/acos-in-your-state.html

Administration on Aging (AOA)
https://aoa.acl.gov

Affordable Care Act (ACA)
https://www.hhs.gov/healthcare/about-the-aca/index.html

Agency for Healthcare Research and Quality (AHRQ)
https://www.ahrq.gov

American Recovery and Reinvestment Act of 2009
https://www.congress.gov/bill/111th-congress/house-bill/1/text

Americans With Disabilities Act of 1990
https://www.eeoc.gov/eeoc/history/35th/1990s/ada.html

Animal and Plant Health Inspection Service (APHIS) / United States Department of Agriculture
https://www.aphis.usda.gov/aphis/home/

Bureau of Labor Statistics (BLS) / United States Bureau of Labor
https://www.bls.gov

CDC: Injury Prevention & Control
https://www.cdc.gov/injury/

Center for Drug Evaluation and Research (CDER) / U.S. Food & Drug Administration
https://www.fda.gov/aboutfda/centersoffices/
officeofmedicalproductsandtobacco/cder/

Centers for Disease Control and Prevention (CDC)
https://www.cdc.gov

Centers for Medicare & Medicaid Services (CMS)
https://www.cms.gov

CMS Innovation Center
https://innovation.cms.gov

Department of Health & Human Services (DHHS)
https://www.hhs.gov

Drug Enforcement Administration
https://www.dea.gov/index.shtml

Emergency Medical Treatment & Labor Act (EMTALA) / Centers for Medicare & Medicaid Services
https://www.cms.gov/regulations-and-guidance/legislation/emtala/

Environmental Protection Agency (EPA) / United States Government
https://www.epa.gov

Eunice Kennedy Shriver National Institute of Child Health and Human Development (NICHD)
https://www.nichd.nih.gov

Facing Addiction in America / The Surgeon General's Report on Alcohol, Drugs, and Health (2016)
https://addiction.surgeongeneral.gov

Facts & Statistics: Roadway Safety Data / U.S. Department of Transportation / Federal Highway Administration
https://safety.fhwa.dot.gov/facts_stats/

Federal Bureau of Investigation (FBI)
https://www.fbi.gov

Food and Drug Administration (FDA) / United States Government
https://www.fda.gov

Federal Trade Commission (FTC) / United States Government
https://www.ftc.gov

Government Accountability Office / United States Government
https://www.gao.gov

Handout on Health: Sports Injuries / National Institute of Arthritis and Musculoskeletal and Skin Diseases
https://www.niams.nih.gov/health_info/sports_injuries/

Health Information Privacy (HIPAA) / U.S. Department of Health & Human Services
https://www.hhs.gov/hipaa/

Insurance Fraud / Federal Bureau of Investigation
https://www.fbi.gov/stats-services/publications/insurance-fraud

Keeping Your Home Safe / An official website of the United States government
https://www.usa.gov/home-safety

Motor Vehicle Crash Deaths / Centers for Disease Control and Prevention
https://www.cdc.gov/vitalsigns/motor-vehicle-safety/

National Cancer Institute
https://www.cancer.gov

National Center for Advancing Translational Sciences (NCATS)
https://ncats.nih.gov

National Center for Complementary and Integrative Health (NCCIH)
https://nccih.nih.gov

National Center for Environmental Health
https://www.cdc.gov/nceh/

National Eye Institute (NEI)
https://www.nei.nih.gov

National Heart, Lung, and Blood Institute (NHLBI)
http://www.nhlbi.nih.gov/index.htm

National Human Genome Research Institute (NHGRI)
https://www.genome.gov

National Institute for Occupational Safety and Health (NIOSH)
https://www.cdc.gov/niosh/

National Institute of Allergy and Infectious Diseases (NIAID)
https://www.niaid.nih.gov

National Institute of Arthritis and Musculoskeletal and Skin Diseases (NIAMS)
https://www.niams.nih.gov

National Institute of Biomedical Imaging and Bioengineering (NIBIB)
https://www.nibib.nih.gov

National Institute of Dental and Craniofacial Research (NIDCR)
https://www.nidcr.nih.gov

National Institute of Diabetes and Digestive and Kidney Diseases (NIDDK)
https://www.niddk.nih.gov

National institute of Environmental Health Sciences (NIEHS)
https://www.niehs.nih.gov

National Institute of General Medical Sciences (NIGMS)
https://www.nigms.nih.gov

National Institute of Mental Health (NIMH)
https://www.nimh.nih.gov

National Institute of Neurological Disorders and Stroke (NINDS)
https://www.ninds.nih.gov

National Institute of Nursing Research (NINR)
https://www.ninr.nih.gov

National Institute on Aging (NIA)
https://www.nia.nih.gov

National Institute on Alcohol Abuse and Alcoholism (NIAAA)
https://www.niaaa.nih.gov

*National Institute on Deafness and Other Communication
Disorders (NIDCD)*
https://www.nidcd.nih.gov

National Institute on Drug Abuse (NIDA)
https://www.drugabuse.gov

*National Institute on Minority Health and Health Disparities
(NIMHD)*
https://www.nimhd.nih.gov

National Institutes of Health (NIH)
https://www.nih.gov

NIH Center for Information Technology
https://www.cit.nih.gov

NIH Center for Scientific Review
https://public.csr.nih.gov

NIH Clinical Center
https://clinicalcenter.nih.gov

Nutrition.gov
https://www.nutrition.gov

Occupational Outlook Handbook (OOH) / U.S. Department of Labor / Bureau of Labor Statistics
https://www.bls.gov/ooh/

Occupational Safety and Health Administration
https://www.osha.gov

Quality Payment Program / CMS
https://qpp.cms.gov

State, Tribal, Local & Territorial Public Health Professionals Gateway
https://www.cdc.gov/stltpublichealth

Surgeon General's Reports on Smoking and Tobacco Use / Centers for Disease Control and Prevention
https://www.cdc.gov/tobacco/data_statistics/sgr/

U.S. National Library of Medicine (NLM)
https://www.nlm.nih.gov

Health Information

Academy of Nutrition and Dietetics
http://www.eatright.org

ALS Association
http://www.alsa.org

Alzheimer's Association
http://www.alz.org

American Association for Visually Handicapped (NAVH)
http://www.navh.org

American Association of Neuromuscular & Electrodiagnostic Medicine (AANEM)
http://www.aanem.org

American Burn Association
http://www.ameriburn.org

American Cancer Society
https://www.cancer.org

American Diabetes Association
http://www.diabetes.org

American Disability Association
http://www.adanet.org

American Fibromyalgia Syndrome Association, Inc. (AFSA)
http://www.afsafund.org

American Geriatrics Society (AGS)
http://www.americangeriatrics.org

American Heart Association (AHA)
http://www.heart.org

American Liver Foundation
http://www.liverfoundation.org

American Lung Association
http://www.lung.org

American Organ Transplant Association (AOTA)
http://www.aotaonline.org

American Parkinson Disease Association (APDA)
https://www.apdaparkinson.org

American Sleep Apnea Association (ASAA)
https://sleepapnea.org

American Stroke Association (ASA)
http://www.strokeassociation.org

America's Health Rankings Annual Report 2016
http://www.americashealthrankings.org

Arthritis Foundation
http://www.arthritis.org

Brain Injury Association of America
http://www.biausa.org

Children with Diabetes Foundation
http://www.cwdfoundation.org

ConsumerMedSafety.org / Protect Yourself From Medication Errors
http://www.consumermedsafety.org

Consumer Rights and Responsibilities / MedlinePlus
https://medlineplus.gov/ency/article/001947.htm

Crohn's & Colitis Foundation
http://www.crohnscolitisfoundation.org

Cleft Palate Foundation (CPF)
http://www.cleftline.org

Defeat Diabetes Foundation
http://www.defeatdiabetes.org

Depression and Bipolar Support Alliance (DBSA)
http://www.dbsalliance.org

Epilepsy Foundation
http://www.epilepsy.com

Erectile Dysfunction (ED)
https://www.erectiledysfunction.com

FACES: The National Craniofacial Association
http://www.faces-cranio.org

Foot.com / Your Foot Health Network
http://www.foot.com/site/

Foundation for Women's Cancer
http://www.thegcf.org

Geriatric Mental Health Foundation (GMHF)
http://www.gmhfonline.org

*Health Care Without Harm / Environmentally Responsible
Healthcare*
https://noharm.org

Institute for Health Metrics and Evaluation
http://www.healthdata.org

Leukemia & Lymphoma Society (LLS)
http://www.lls.org

Material Safety Data Sheets / Where To Find On The Internet
http://www.ilpi.com/msds/

Medscape.com
http://www.medscape.com

Mental Health America (MHA)
http://www.mentalhealthamerica.net

Modern Healthcare / The Leader In Healthcare Business News, Research & Data
http://www.modernhealthcare.com

Muscular Dystrophy Association (MDA)
https://www.mda.org

National Association for Down Syndrome (NADS)
http://www.nads.org

National Children's Cancer Society
https://thenccs.org

National Council on Aging: Center for Healthy Aging
https://www.ncoa.org/center-for-healthy-aging/

National Hemophilia Foundation (NHF)
https://www.hemophilia.org

National Kidney Cancer Association
https://www.kidneycancer.org

National Kidney Foundation
https://www.kidney.org

National Multiple Sclerosis Society
http://www.nationalmssociety.org/What-is-MS

National Osteoporosis Foundation
https://www.nof.org

National Parkinson Foundation (NPF)
http://www.parkinson.org

National Psoriasis Foundation/USA
https://www.psoriasis.org/about-psoriasis

National Safety Council (NSC)
http://www.nsc.org

Prevention Hub
http://preventionhub.org/en

Robert Wood Johnson Foundation (RWJF)
http://www.rwjf.org

Spine-Health.com
http://www.spine-health.com

Miscellaneous Health-Related Sites

A Census of Actively Licensed Physicians in the United States, 2014
https://www.fsmb.org/Media/Default/PDF/Census/2014census.pdf

Bill & Melinda Gates Foundation
http://www.gatesfoundation.org

CARB-X / Promoter of public-private partnerships against antibiotic resistance
http://carb-x.org/

Chan Zuckerberg Initiative
https://chanzuckerberg.com

Henry J. Kaiser Family Foundation
http://kff.org

Immunization, Vaccines and Biologicals / World Health Organization (WHO)
http://www.who.int/immunization/diseases/en/

International Agency for Research on Cancer (IARC)
http://www.iarc.fr

The National Academies of Sciences/Engineering/Medicine
http://national-academies.org

Origins and Future of Accountable Care Organizations / Leavitt
https://www.brookings.edu/wp-content/uploads/2016/06/Impact-of-Accountable-CareOrigins-052015.pdf

Pan American Health Organization (PAHO)
http://www.paho.org/hq/

Patient-Centered Primary Care Collaborative
https://www.pcpcc.org/about

The Patient-Centered Medical Home / Primary Care Progress
http://www.primarycareprogress.org/pcmh

World Health Organization (WHO)
http://www.who.int/en/

Most-Popular Health Websites - April 2017

WebMD
http://www.webmd.com

National Institutes of Health
https://www.nih.gov

Yahoo! Health
https://www.yahoo.com/beauty/tagged/health

Mayo Clinic
http://www.mayoclinic.org

MedicineNet.com
http://www.medicinenet.com/script/main/hp.asp

Drugs.com
https://www.drugs.com

Everyday Health
http://www.everydayhealth.com

HealthGrades
https://www.healthgrades.com

HealthLine
http://www.healthline.com

Mercola
http://www.mercola.com

Health
http://www.health.com

Mind Body Green
https://www.mindbodygreen.com

Medscape
http://www.medscape.com

RxList
http://www.rxlist.com/script/main/hp.asp

Medical News Today
http://www.medicalnewstoday.com

Patient Safety

Cautious Patient Foundation
http://cautiouspatient.org

Defining Medical Error / US National Library of Medicine
https://www.ncbi.nlm.nih.gov/pmc/articles/PMC3211566/

Institute for Healthcare Improvement
http://www.ihi.org/Topics/PatientSafety/Pages/default.aspx

National Patient Safety Foundation
http://www.npsf.org

Patient Safety / HealthCatalyst
https://www.healthcatalyst.com/improving-patient-safety-and-quality-in-healthcare

Patient Safety / MedlinePlus
https://medlineplus.gov/patientsafety.html

Patient Safety / World Health Organization
http://www.who.int/patientsafety/en/

The Joint Commission on Patient Safety
https://www.jointcommission.org/topics/patient_safety.aspx

What Is Patient Safety? / Leapfrog Hospital Safety Grade
http://www.hospitalsafetygrade.org/what-is-patient-safety_m

Professional & Industry Associations & Societies:

American Academy of Allergy, Asthma & Immunology
http://www.aaaai.org

American Academy of Child & Adolescent Psychiatry (AACAP)
http://www.aacap.org

American Academy of Cosmetic Surgery
http://www.cosmeticsurgery.org

American Academy of Dermatology (AAD)
https://www.aad.org

American Academy of Emergency Medicine (AAEM)
http://www.aaem.org

American Academy of Family Physicians (AAFP)
http://www.aafp.org

American Academy of Neurology (AAN)
https://www.aan.com

American Academy of Ophthalmology (AAO)
https://www.aao.org

American Academy of Oral and Maxillofacial Radiology (AAOMR)
https://www.aaomr.org

American Academy of Orthopaedic Surgeons (AAOS)
http://www.aaos.org

American Academy of Otolaryngology - Head and Heck Surgery
http://www.entnet.org

American Academy of Pain Medicine (AAPM)
http://www.painmed.org

American Academy of Pediatrics (AAP)
https://www.aap.org

American Academy of Physical Medicine and Rehabilitation (AAPM&R)
http://www.aapmr.org

American Academy of Physician Assistants (AAPA)
https://www.aapa.org

American Academy of Professional Coders (AAPC)
https://www.aapc.com

American Association for Cancer Research (AACR)
http://www.aacr.org

American Association for Geriatric Psychiatry (AAGP)
http://www.aagponline.org

American Association for Respiratory Care (AARC)
https://www.aarc.org

American Association for the Study of Liver Diseases (AASLD)
http://www.aasld.org

American Association for Women Radiologists (AAWR)
http://www.aawr.org

American Association of Blood Banks (AABB)
http://www.aabb.org

American Association of Certified Orthoptists (AACO)
http://orthoptics.org

American Association of Clinical Endocrinologists (AACE)
https://www.aace.com

American Association of Gynecologic Laparoscopists (AAGL)
http://www.aagl.org

American Association of Hip and Knee Surgeons (AAHKS)
http://www.aahks.org

American Association of Immunologists (AAI)
http://www.aai.org

American Association of Neurological Surgeons (AANS)
http://www.aans.org

American Association of Neuroscience Nurses (AANN)
http://aann.org

American Association of Nurse Practitioners (AANP)
https://www.aanp.org

American Association of Pharmaceutical Scientists (AAPS)
http://www.aaps.org/default.aspx

American Association of Physicists in Medicine (AAPM)
http://www.aapm.org

American Association of Plastic Surgeons (AAPS)
http://www.aaps1921.org

American Chiropractic Association (ACA)
https://www.acatoday.org

American Clinical Neurophysiology Society (ACNS)
http://www.acns.org

American College of Cardiology
http://www.acc.org

American College of Chest Physicians (ACCP)
http://www.chestnet.org

American College of Emergency Physicians (ACEP)
https://www.acep.org

American College of Healthcare Executives (ACHE)
http://ache.org

American College of Managed Care Medicine, Inc.
http://www.acmcm.org

American College of Medical Genetics and Genomics (ACMG)
https://www.acmg.net

American College of Nuclear Physicians (ACNP)
http://www.acnmonline.org

American College of Physicians (ACP)
https://www.acponline.org

American College of Preventive Medicine (ACPM)
http://www.acpm.org

American College of Radiation Oncology (ACRO)
https://www.acro.org

American College of Radiology (ACR)
https://www.acr.org

American College of Rheumatology (ACR)
http://www.rheumatology.org

American College of Surgeons (ACS)
https://www.facs.org

American Congress of Obstetricians and Gynecologists (ACOG)
http://www.acog.org

American Dental Association (ADA)
http://www.ada.org/en

American Dental Education Association (ADEA)
http://www.adea.org

American Dermatological Association
http://www.amer-derm-assn.org

American Epilepsy Society
https://www.aesnet.org

American Genetic Association (AGA)
http://www.theaga.org

American Health Information Management Association (AHIMA)
http://www.ahima.org

American Health Insurance Plans (AHIP)
https://www.ahip.org

American Healthcare Radiology Administrators (AHRA)
http://www.ahra.org

American Hospital Association (AHA)
http://www.aha.org

American Institute of Ultrasound in Medicine (AIUM)
http://www.aium.org

American Liver Foundation (ALF)
http://www.liverfoundation.org

American Medical Informatics Association (AMIA)
https://www.amia.org

American Medical Women's Association (AMWA)
https://www.amwa-doc.org

American Medical Group Association (AMGA)
http://www.amga.org

American Medical Association (AMA)
https://www.ama-assn.org

American Neurological Association (ANA)
https://myana.org

American Nuclear Society (ANS)
http://www.ans.org

American Nurses Association (ANA)
http://www.nursingworld.org

American Orthopaedic Society for Sports Medicine (AOSSM)
http://www.sportsmed.org/aossmimis

American Osteopathic Association (AOA)
http://www.osteopathic.org

American Osteopathic College of Radiology (AOCR)
http://www.aocr.org

American Pharmaceutical Association (APhA)
http://www.aphanet.org

American Physical Therapy Association (APTA)
http://www.apta.org

American Podiatric Medical Association (APMA)
http://www.apma.org

American Psychiatric Association (APA)
https://www.psychiatry.org

American Psychological Association (APA)
http://www.apa.org

American Public Health Association (APHA)
https://www.apha.org

American Radium Society (ARS)
https://www.americanradiumsociety.org

American Registry of Diagnostic Medical Sonographers (ARDMS)
http://www.ardms.org/Pages/default.aspx

American Registry of Radiologic Technologists (ARRT)
https://www.arrt.org

American Rhinologic Society (ARS)
https://www.american-rhinologic.org

American Roentgen Ray Society (ARRS)
http://www.arrs.org

American Society for Biochemistry and Molecular Biology (ASBMB)
http://www.asbmb.org

American Society for Bone & Mineral Research (ASBMR)
http://www.asbmr.org

American Society for Cell Biology (ASCB)
http://www.ascb.org

American Society for Clinical Investigation (ASCI)
https://www.the-asci.org

American Society for Clinical Pathology (ASCP)
https://www.ascp.org/content

American Society for Dermatologic Surgery (ASDS)
https://www.asds.net

American Society for Gastrointestinal Endoscopy (ASGE)
https://www.asge.org

American Society for Microbiology (ASM)
http://www.asm.org

American Society for Nutrition (ASN)
http://www.nutrition.org

*American Society for Therapeutic Radiology and Oncology
(ASTRO)*
https://www.astro.org/home/

American Society of Addiction Medicine (ASAM)
http://www.asam.org

American Society of Anesthesiologists
http://www.asahq.org

American Society of Cataract and Refractive Surgery (ASCRS)
http://www.ascrs.org

American Society of Clinical Oncology (ASCO)
http://www.asco.org

American Society of Echocardiography (ASE)
http://asecho.org

American Society of Emergency Radiology (ASER)
http://www.erad.org

American Society of Head and Neck Radiology (ASHNR)
http://ashnr.org

American Society of Health-System Pharmacists (ASHP)
https://www.ashp.org

American Society of Hematology (ASH)
http://www.hematology.org

American Society of Hypertension, Inc. (ASH)
http://www.ash-us.org

American Society of Nephrology (ASN)
https://www.asn-online.org

American Society of Neuroimaging (ASN)
https://www.asnweb.org

American Society of Neuroradiology (ASNR)
https://www.asnr.org

American Society of Nuclear Cardiology (ASNC)
http://www.asnc.org

American Society of Ophthalmic Plastic & Reconstructive Surgery (ASOPRS)
https://www.asoprs.org

American Society of Plastic Surgeons (ASPS)
https://www.plasticsurgery.org

American Society of Radiologic Technologists (ASRT)
https://www.asrt.org

American Society of Transplant Surgeons (ASTS)
http://asts.org

American Society of Transplantation (AST)
https://www.myast.org

American Society of Tropical Medicine & Hygiene (ASTMH)
http://www.astmh.org

American Speech-language-Hearing Association
http://www.asha.org

American Spinal Injury Association (ASIA)
http://asia-spinalinjury.org

American Telemedicine Association (ATA)
http://www.americantelemed.org/home

American Thoracic Society (ATS)
http://www.thoracic.org

American Thyroid Association (ATA)
http://www.thyroid.org

American Tinnitus Association (ATA)
https://www.ata.org

American Urological Association (AUA)
http://www.auanet.org

Association for Healthcare Documentation Integrity (AHDI)
http://www.ahdionline.org

Association for Humanistic Psychology (AHP)
https://www.ahpweb.org

Association of American Medical Colleges (AAMC)
https://www.aamc.org

Association of Genetic Technologists, Inc. (AGT)
http://www.agt-info.org

Association of Military Osteopathic Physicians and Surgeons (AMOPS)
http://amops.org

Association of Oncology Social Work (AOSW)
http://www.aosw.org

Association of Operating Room Nurses (AORN)
http://www.aorn.org

Association of Organ Procurement Organizations (AOPO)
http://www.aopo.org

Association of Pediatric Hematology/Oncology Nurses (APHON)
http://aphon.org

Association of Physician Assistants in Obstetrics and Gynecology (APAOG)
http://www.paobgyn.org

Association of Professors of Gynecology and Obstetrics (APGO)
https://www.apgo.org

Association of Program Directors in Endocrinology, Diabetes, and Metabolism (APDEM)
http://www.apdem.org

Association of Residents in Radiation Oncology (ARRO)
https://www.astro.org/arro.aspx

Association of Telemedicine Service Providers (ATSP)
http://www.atsp.org

Association of University Radiologists (AUR)
http://www.aur.org

Association of Vascular and Interventional Radiographers (AVIR)
http://www.avir.org

Behavior Genetics Association (BGA)
http://bga.org

Central Association of Obstetricians & Gynecologists (CAOG)
http://www.caog.org

Cleveland Clinic / Health Library
https://my.clevelandclinic.org/health

College of American Pathologists (CAP)
http://www.cap.org

Colon Cancer Alliance
https://www.ccalliance.org

Council of Medical Specialty Societies (CMSS)
https://cmss.org

Dermatology Nurses' Association (DNA)
https://www.dnanurse.org

Emergency Medicine Residents' Association (EMRA)
https://www.emra.org

Emergency Nurses Association (ENA)
https://www.ena.org

Endocrine Fellows Foundation (EFF)
http://www.endocrinefellows.org

Endocrine Society
https://www.endocrine.org

Federation of American Societies for Experimental Biology (FASEB)
http://www.faseb.org

Healthcare Business Management Association (HBMA)
http://www.hbma.org

Heart Rhythm Society (HRS)
http://www.hrsonline.org

Infectious Diseases Society of America (IDSA)
http://www.idsociety.org

International Anaplastology Association
http://www.anaplastology.org

International Association of Physicians in AIDS Care (IAPAC)
http://www.iapac.org

Mayo Clinic / Patient Care and Health Information
http://www.mayoclinic.org/patient-care-and-health-information

Medical Group Management Association (MGMA)
http://www.mgma.com

Musculoskeletal Ultrasound Society
http://musoc.com

National Association of Health Data Organizations (NAHDO)
https://www.nahdo.org

National Center for Interprofessional Practice and Education
https://nexusipe.org/informing/about-national-center

National Foundation for Infectious Diseases (NFID)
http://www.nfid.org

National Organization for Rare Disorders (NORD)
https://rarediseases.org

National Rural Health Association (NRHA)
https://www.ruralhealthweb.org

National Student Nurses Association (NSNA)
http://www.nsna.org

North American Association of Central Cancer Registries (NAACCR)
https://www.naaccr.org

North American Society for Cardiac Imaging (NASCI)
http://www.nasci.org

North American Spinal Society (NASS)
https://www.spine.org

Nuclear Medicine Technology Certification Board (NMTCB)
http://www.nmtcb.org

Obesity Medicine Association
https://obesitymedicine.org

Pharmaceutical Research and Manufacturers of America (PhRMA)
http://www.phrma.org

Prostate Cancer Foundation (PCF)
https://www.pcf.org

Radiation Research Society
http://www.radres.org

Radiation Therapy Oncology Group (RTOG)
https://www.rtog.org

Radiological Society of North America (RSNA)
http://www.rsna.org

Radiology Business Management Association (RBMA)
http://www.rbma.org

Society for Academic Emergency Medicine (SAEM)
http://www.saem.org

Society for the Advancement of Women's Imaging (SAWI)
http://www.sawi.org

Society for Cardiac Angiography and Interventions (SCAI)
http://www.scai.org

Society for Cardiovascular Magnetic Resonance
http://scmr.org

Society for Endocrinology
http://www.endocrinology.org

Society for Investigative Dermatology (SID)
http://www.sidnet.org

Society for Neuroscience (SFN)
http://www.sfn.org

Society for Pediatric Pathology (SPP)
http://www.spponline.org

Society of American Gastrointestinal and Endoscopic Surgeons (SAGES)
https://www.sages.org

Society of Breast Imaging (SBI)
http://www.sbi-online.org

Society of Computed Body Tomography and Magnetic Resource (SCBT/MR)
http://www.scbtmr.org

Society of Critical Care Medicine
http://www.sccm.org

Society of Diagnostic Medical Sonographers (SDMS)
http://www.sdms.org

Society of Gastroenterology Nurses and Associates, Inc. (SGNA)
https://www.sgna.org

Society of General Internal Medicine (SGIM)
http://www.sgim.org

Society of Gynecologic Oncology (SGO)
https://www.sgo.org

Society of Interventional Radiology
http://www.scvir.org

Society of Nuclear Medicine and Molecular Imaging (SNM / MI)
http://www.snmmi.org

Society of Radiology Oncology Administrators (SROA)
https://www.sroa.org

Society of Skeletal Radiology (SSR)
https://skeletalrad.org

Society of Thoracic Radiology (STR)
http://thoracicrad.org

Society of Thoracic Surgeons (STS)
http://www.sts.org

Society to Improve Diagnosis in Medicine
http://www.improvediagnosis.org

Teratology Society
https://www.teratology.org

United Network for Organ Sharing (UNOS)
https://www.unos.org

U.S. Pharmacopeial Convention (USPC)
http://www.usp.org

Rating / Ranking / Review Sites:

Angie's List / Health
https://www.angieslist.com/health/

CareDash / Find, Compare, and Review Doctors
https://www.caredash.com

Dr. Social
http://drsocial.org

HealthGrades.com
https://www.healthgrades.com

Hospital Compare / Medicare.gov
https://www.medicare.gov/hospitalcompare/search.html?

Hospital Ratings / Consumer Reports
http://www.consumerreports.org/health/hospitals/ratings

Leapfrog Hospital Safety Grade
http://www.hospitalsafetygrade.org

Rate MDs
https://www.ratemds.com

The Leapfrog Group
http://www.leapfroggroup.org

Nursing Home Compare / Medicare.gov
https://www.medicare.gov/nursinghomecompare/search.html

Top Doctors
http://www.topdrz.com

U.S. News & World Report's 2017 Best Medical Schools
https://www.usnews.com/best-graduate-schools/top-medical-schools?int=a4d609

U.S. News & World Report's 2016-2017 Best Hospitals Honor Roll
https://www.usnews.com/info/blogs/press-room/articles/2016-08-02/us-news-announces-the-201617-best-hospitals

Vitals.com
http://www.vitals.com

WebMD Physician Directory
http://doctor.webmd.com

Yelp
https://www.yelp.com

ZocDocs
https://www.zocdoc.com

PREVIEW.

SUCCESSFUL PATIENT

Step-By-Step Strategies

To Get The Health Care You Need

by Linda Hewitt

Coming October 31, 2017

Chapter One.

No One Expects The Unexpected

No one expects the unexpected.

It sounds like a truism so obvious as to be beyond cliché. But real life is a lot more cliché than most of us want to admit.

So, this being real life, let's concede *No one expects the unexpected*, and get to the point of this book, which begins with a simple observation. For most of us, good health is rarely noticed, and bad health strikes us as so *not* what our lives are supposed to be about that its appearance often triggers a bizarre combination of panic and cluelessness.

Maybe some of it is due to the speed with which things can happen. There you are, lunchtime, busy city sidewalk, everybody going about their business, you're wondering whether you've got time to order off the menu, and suddenly something happens. Maybe you start seeing double and the top of your head feels as if it's about to dissolve. Maybe that niggling prickling in your side that's been bothering you for months turns into pain too intense to be ignored. Maybe a fellow pedestrian in a hurry brushes by, making you lose your balance, and you actually hear your arm snap when you hit the sidewalk. Maybe a car jumps the curb and hits you. From one breath to another, you have ceased being you "the butcher, baker, candlestick maker" and become a *patient*. Out of the blue, you have taken the first step that leads into The Provider Universe, that large, sometimes amorphous conglomeration of doctors, nurses, dentists, therapists, hospitals, ambulatory care facilities, and all the other occupations and entities that work together to provide health care to residents of the United States. That first step, incidentally, is rarely reversible. Once in The Provider Universe, you are likely to remain there for at least a while.

Equally horrifying is when you're fine and it's someone you care about who suddenly turns to you in the middle of dinner or at a ball game and says, "Honey, I've got a strange pain. I think I need to go to the emergency room."

Either way, you are about to enter a world whose resemblance to your usual surroundings and routine is only superficial. Furthermore, it's a world in which momentum develops with the seeming inevitability of a tidal wave, and — whether patient or advocate for patient — you find yourself being swept along in a way that the normal, sensible you would not think possible.

There are tests, diagnoses, and procedures in facilities that manage to seem both reassuring and vaguely ominous. A series of professionally pleasant people appear, perform specific duties, and then disappear, many never to be seen again. Test results arrive, interpreted by yet other professionals. You are told certain things about what is wrong. The doctor pronounces the recommended course of treatment as if it is written in stone. Even as your providers go through the motions of acquiring your "informed consent" there is clearly an assumption that you are indeed willing to proceed simply because they have told you it is the next step.

You are now on a health-care treadmill, and oftentimes may make decisions without quite realizing that you've done so, what will follow, or that there were other options.

Each stage of your progression through the system, you may have a sense that everyone but you has authority and control, that there is some underlying pattern affecting care in ways you don't quite understand, and that patients are almost incidental to the process. Worst of all, you may even have a sneaking suspicion that, somewhere, there is a better way to address the problem — a more-expert doctor, a more-advanced treatment regimen, a way to get better faster.

Then, whatever the outcome, you may find yourself confronted by a slew of financial issues, some dreaded, some of which you had no idea were coming.

Being sick or injured is bad enough. You don't need complications — no pun intended — especially when they're caused by lack of knowledge.

I keep saying "you" when what I'm talking about is the way the health-provider community (of which I'm a big fan, incidentally) managed to make me feel at times, especially when my seemingly healthy and well-insured husband had emergency heart procedures. But that's me. Maybe you're immune to uncertainty in unfamiliar surroundings, are not bothered by having to repeat medical procedures unnecessarily, and have a laissez-faire attitude toward money and time. If so, go no further — your knack for spontaneity will stand you in good stead when the unexpected happens. If, however, you share my sense that it would be useful to prepare for success as a patient or advocate, then this book's for you.

Let me say up front that this is not a book of complaints, because I consider our experiences to have been generally positive and our providers excellent. Nor does it give medical, legal, or financial advice. I've worked in insurance and, as a consultant, written and researched extensively about health care and related issues for corporate clients, but that doesn't make me a medical professional, a lawyer, or an accountant. Nor is it a cry for reform — that issue is too complex and fluid to be addressed by a non-professional in a relatively modest book. Nor does it attempt to address possible changes in health care that may or may not result from political action.

Rather, *Successful Patient* focuses on the development of a personal strategy for navigating The Provider Universe as it exists today, a strategy based on individual priorities and leveraging options to get the right care. In essence, this is the book I wish I'd had access to while waiting outside one emergency room or other.

The book consists of five parts:

◊ **Part One.** *The Patient Experience considers the evolution of medicine to its current, near-miraculous state, and takes a quick look at the two personal health episodes that prompted a lot of research and the writing of this book.*

◊ **Part Two.** *The Need For A Personal Health-Care Strategy summarizes the argument for devising a strategy in order to overcome the obstacles presented by The Provider Universe and patients themselves and also examines what strategy should include.*

◊ **Part Three.** *Step-by-Step Strategy goes through the development of a personal strategy in detail, incorporating twelve stages that begin with things you can do "in advance of need" and moving forward through the system most patients will encounter.*

◊ **Part Four.** *The Money Thing summarizes some of the financial considerations that can pop up and what you can do to handle them in the way that works best for you.*

◊ **Part Five.** *Resources provides a list of online resources that you* *may find useful as you develop and work your strategy.*

The bottom line is that — even though The Provider Universe exists to serve patients — its focus is more than a little fragmented at the moment by an impressive combination of medical advances, quality initiatives, patient self-determination, and attempts to impose cost controls. In the long term, all of this should improve outcomes. In the short term, this is not an environment in which we want to leave to chance anything we as patients value or need.

Having a strategy won't guarantee that when the unexpected happens and we become patients we will get everything we want, but it'll make it a lot more likely that we get what we need from a system that, when functioning at its highest and best level, is literally capable of performing miracles.

END OF PREVIEW

COLOPHON

The body copy of this book is set in Minion Pro, designed in 1990 by Robert Slimbach for Adobe. The headings are in Britannic Bold, a digital version of a design originally created in 1901 by the Wagner & Schmidt foundry of Leipzig, Germany. Resources list is in Minion Pro Semibold Italic and Arial. The creation program was Adobe's InDesign, The cover and book design were by Robert Hewitt, executed in Photoshop. The printing method of the book was (1) for the trade paperback, Print-On-Demand from CreateSpace and (2) for the hardback, Ingram Spark.

A Warning
With apologies to that long-ago scribe in Nineveh who thusly protected the tablet on which he carved his words, as well as to those patient monks who did not have the benefit of digital typesetting, here's a nod to tradition with a book curse.

They who tear apart this book or dowse it in water or burn it in flame or atomize it with Vril or destroy or misuse it in any other manner or fashion (including non-permitted use and/or unacknowledged appropriation of its contents by any means) may Benjamin Franklin, Thomas Jefferson, Alexander Hamilton, Isaiah Thomas, Hannah Crocker, William Bentley, John Jacob Astor, John Codman, James Lenox, Samuel J. Tilden, Andrew Carnegie, Andrew Mellon and all the other gods of the library and the gods of all dedicated readers curse them with a curse that cannot be relieved, terrible and merciless, as long as they live, may the gods let their names be known far and wide as desecrators of the written word, enemies to knowledge, perverters of simple pleasures, exploiters of the laborer, unworthy to be allowed further access to the hallowed precincts of shared thought through time.

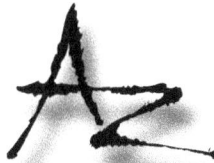

ArbeitenZeit Media

www.ingramcontent.com/pod-product-compliance
Lightning Source LLC
Chambersburg PA
CBHW081413270326
41931CB00015B/3262